Consulting with Pediatricians

Psychological Perspectives

Issues in Clinical Child Psychology

Series Editors: **Michael C. Roberts,** *University of Kansas–Lawrence, Kansas*
Lizette Peterson, *University of Missouri–Columbia, Missouri*

BEHAVIORAL ASPECTS OF PEDIATRIC BURNS
Edited by Kenneth J. Tarnowski

CHILDREN AND DISASTERS
Edited by Conway F. Saylor

CONSULTING WITH PEDIATRICIANS: Psychological Perspectives
Dennis Drotar

HANDBOOK OF DEPRESSION IN CHILDREN AND ADOLESCENTS
Edited by William M. Reynolds and Hugh F. Johnston

INTERNATIONAL HANDBOOK OF PHOBIC AND ANXIETY DISORDERS IN CHILDREN AND ADOLESCENTS
Edited by Thomas H. Ollendick, Neville J. King, and William Yule

MENTAL HEALTH INTERVENTIONS WITH PRESCHOOL CHILDREN
Robert D. Lyman and Toni L. Hembree-Kigin

A Continuation Order Plan is available for this series. A continuation order will bring delivery of each new volume immediately upon publication. Volumes are billed only upon actual shipment. For further information please contact the publisher.

Consulting with Pediatricians

Psychological Perspectives

DENNIS DROTAR

Case Western Reserve University
School of Medicine
Cleveland, Ohio

With Contributions by

PEGGY CRAWFORD
CARIN CUNNINGHAM
LINDA K. HURLEY
SUSAN L. ROSENTHAL

PLENUM PRESS • NEW YORK AND LONDON

Library of Congress Cataloging-in-Publication Data

On file

ISBN 0-306-44935-8

A Division of Plenum Publishing Corporation
233 Spring Street, New York, N. Y. 10013

10 9 8 7 6 5 4 3 2 1

Printed in the United States of America

To Peg, my wife and companion,
whose steadfast support, understanding, and commitment
have taught me the true meaning of collaboration and love

Preface

This book is based on the assumption that collaborative interdisciplinary efforts in clinical practice, research, and training will produce more informed professionals, more effective psychological services, and greater advances in scientific knowledge than will solitary professional efforts. This idea is not new; others have also held it (Anderson, 1930; Kagan, 1965; Richmond, 1967; Wright, 1967). However, this volume was stimulated in part by my continuing concern that the level and quality of collaboration between psychologists and physicians have not always lived up to the initial promise that was outlined by the founders of pediatric psychology partly because it can be such a difficult enterprise (Drotar, 1983, 1993).

In many respects, interprofessional tensions and lost collaborative opportunities are understandable when one considers the obstacles to interdisciplinary collaboration (Drotar, 1993; Friedman, 1985). Many physicians, including pediatricians, have a limited exposure to collaborative activities with other professions, including psychologists, and are not familiar with the full range of their potential contributions (Davidson, 1988). This limited exposure is a two-way street: Because psychologists are trained almost exclusively by other psychologists, they are not especially conversant with pediatricians' unique professional strengths and knowledge base (Levine, 1990), their needs and expectations concerning collaboration (Davidson, 1988), or their work-related stressors and strains (Good & Good, 1989). Consequently, many pediatricians and psychologists do not reap the potential benefits of such work for practice, teaching, and research. Others have difficulty setting clear, realistic expectations for the goals and outcomes of interprofessional work. Some professionals may become so frustrated with the problems inherent in collaboration that they limit or even abandon their cooperative work in favor of professional isolation.

Other salient features of the collaborative process also contribute to difficulties in learning and practicing collaboration. Collaboration is not the exclusive province of any single profession. Rather, its essence lies in the *relationship* among individuals in different professions or between professional groups. However, issues that arise in the relationships among professional disciplines generally are not addressed in standards of professional practice and ethics. Such issues as which profession is responsible for initiating or maintaining collaborative patient care, research, or teaching; the specific roles and responsibilities in collaborative work; and standards of evaluation of collaborative activities have not been thoroughly considered.

The relatively limited focus on interdisciplinary collaboration in professional training and practice has been paralleled by inconsistent writings and research on this topic. Moreover, publications have been scattered across many different professional journals and books. Published work has not described the full range of collaborative activities, showcased new and innovative efforts, or provided a vehicle to learn from those who have struggled through difficulties to forge successful collaborative ties. Yet interdisciplinary collaboration remains a highly prized, professionally relevant activity for psychologists. In our recent survey, pediatric psychologists rated collaboration with pediatric colleagues as among the highest sources of their work-related satisfaction (Drotar, Sturm, Eckerle, & White, 1993). Moreover, the continued development of the field of pediatric psychology will depend on the quality of psychologists' collaborative efforts, not only with pediatricians but also with other professionals (Drotar, 1991).

My hope is that this volume will facilitate the collaborative efforts of professionals, but especially that of psychologists and pediatricians in medical settings, by presenting a comprehensive view of the potential and pitfalls of collaborative work in the 1990s. This work distills personal experiences drawn from more than 20 years of collaborative clinical work, research, and teaching with pediatricians in medical settings and in professional organizations. Starting in 1966 with my training in a graduate-level pediatric psychology program at the University of Iowa, which was a collaborative effort among psychologists and pediatricians (Routh, 1969), and continuing until the present, I have been involved in some type of collaboration with pediatricians throughout my professional career. Although these collaborative roads have not always been smooth, I remain convinced of the worth of the journey. This book summarizes some of the lessons I have learned. My hope is that it will help others negotiate their own collaborative paths a little easier.

The prospect of writing this book has provided me with an opportunity to reflect on the field of pediatric psychology and on the many individuals who have taught me and provided support. Pediatric psychology has been shaped into the vibrant field it is today by the personal qualities of practitioners, teachers, and researchers in this field. This book did not spring *de novo* but reflects a long history of shared experiences with a large number of colleagues. I have been very fortunate to have worked with outstanding clinical and research mentors and to have observed their professional collaborations. A short list of such mentors includes Jane Anderson, Bruce Cushna, Gail Gardner, Camille Hanlon, Dick Lanyon, Joe Lord, Don Routh, and Ira Semler. As a postdoctoral fellow, I had the opportunity to train with Gail Gardner in a newly developed pediatric psychology service in the Department of Pediatrics at the University of Colorado Medical Center. Starting with his mentorship at Iowa and continuing to the present, my professional association and friendship with Don Routh have been a source of inspiration and influence as they have for so many others in the field of pediatric psychology. I have not been able to figure how Don accomplishes all he does, but I know it has something to do with hard work and a lot with character.

I have learned a great deal about collaborating with pediatricians from psychologist colleagues, especially Gary Mesibov, Michael Roberts, Carolyn Schroeder, Brian Stabler, Terry Stancin, Sue White, and Ken Whitt. A while ago, Brian, Ken, and I spent some time putting together a traveling road show (or was it a workshop?) concerning consultation that helped to shape some of my ideas (Stabler, Whitt, & Drotar, 1979).

My relationships with colleagues in pediatrics, nursing, and social work have been a source of continuing satisfaction and professional stimulation. Some of these colleagues have included Tom Boat, Peggy Crawford, Bill Dahms, Doug Kerr, Mary Ann Ganofsky, Laura Guay, Nancy Irvin, John Kennell, Marshall Klaus, Sally Lambert, Marilyn Litvene, Suddesh Makker, Howard Maltz, Leroy Matthews, Karen Olness, Bob Stern, and Max Wiznitzer. In addition, my colleagues in the Research Consortium in Childhood Chronic Illness and Society for Behavioral Pediatrics and Task Force for Coding of Mental Health in Children have provided gratifying opportunities for collaboration that have transcended institutional walls.

Finally, my work in training psychologists to work with pediatricians in clinical work and research has been a continuing and positive force in my own career. These students, interns, and fellows have included Laura Basili, Karen Berkoff, Beth Anne Bull, Barbara Boat, Marcy Bush, Carin Cunningham, Steve Evans, Yonit Hoffman, Carol Fitzpatrick, Carolyn Ievers, Carol Kucia, Tonya Mizell, Jack Nassau, Nancy Peterson, Charisse Peoples, Sean Phipps, Suzanne Powell, Lois Rifner, Ron Saletsky, Lynn Singer, and Lynne Sturm. They and others like them will shape the future of collaborative work.

DENNIS DROTAR

Acknowledgments

I would like to acknowledge the hard work and dedication of several people whose much-appreciated word-processing help and expertise helped to make this book possible: Kathy Gill, Claire Svet, and most especially Annette Waters, who did the majority of the word processing. I'm sure that they were especially happy to see the completion of this work.

I would also like to acknowledge the help of Michael Roberts and Lizette Peterson, who stimulated this volume (got me into this!) and provided helpful feedback and support.

Contents

Introduction 1
Consulting with Physicians Other Than Pediatricians 3

Part I

Chapter 1. Evolution of Collaboration among Psychologists and Pediatricians: A Brief History 7

Development of Pediatrics in the United States 7
Early Developments in Collaboration 9
The Emergence of Developmental and Behavioral Pediatrics 11
Developments in Pediatrician/Psychologist Collaboration 13
  Early Clinical Collaborations 13
  Early Collaborative Teaching and Training Efforts 13
Early Visions of Collaboration: Psychologists' Views 15
Modern Growth of Collaboration 16

Chapter 2. Models of Collaborative Activities and Influences 19

Description of Collaborative Activities 19
  Goal or Content 20
  Settings 20
  Characteristics of Collaborators 21
  Outcomes 22
  Relationship Characteristics and Outcome 22
  Stages of Collaborative Relationships 22
Models of Collaboration/Consultation in Pediatric Psychology ... 23
  Independent Functions Model 23
  Indirect Consultation Model 24

Collaborative Team Model 26
Systems Approach 26
Influences on Collaborative Outcomes 28
Beliefs and Expectations Concerning Collaboration 28
Collaborative Skills and Knowledge 31
Situational Incentives and Constraints 31
Importance of Professional Socialization 32
Implications: Enhancing Collaborative Success 32

Chapter 3. Consultation and Collaboration in Primary Care Settings 35

Referral Problems and Services in Primary Care Settings 36
Consultation in Primary Care Academic Medical Settings 37
Structuring Service Delivery 37
Teaching Pediatricians in Primary Care Settings 38
Guidelines for Clinical Consultation in Primary Care Settings 40
Clarifying the Referrral Request 40
Structuring Referral Procedures 40
Discussing the Referral with Family Members 41
Giving Feedback to Pediatricians 42
Other Consultation Methods 43
Psychological Consultation in Community Pediatric Practice: Schroeder and Her Colleagues' Collaborative Practice Model 44
Collaborative Research in Primary Care Settings 46

Chapter 4. Consultation and Collaboration in Pediatric Inpatient Settings 49

Referral Problems/Services in Inpatient Settings 49
Intervention and Follow-Up 50
Guidelines for Clinical Consultation with Hospitalized Children Clarifying Referral Requests 51
Communicating with Multiple Staff 53
Informing the Child and Parents 53
Actions and Responsibilities in Psychological Consultation 54
Psychological Assessment 54
Communication to Staff 55
Giving Direct Feedback to Staff 56
Feedback to Parents and Child 56
Arranging Follow-Up 57
Specialized Consultation Procedures 57

Structuring Collaborative Case Reviews and Planning 58
Implementing a Collaborative Case Review 58
Follow-Up 59
Implementing Ongoing Case Reviews 59
Liaison with Other Professional Staff 61
Group Problem Solving to Enhance Policy and Practice 61
Teaching through Case Reviews 62

Chapter 5. Collaborating with Other Professions in Pediatric Settings 65

Need for a Broad-Based Interdisciplinary Collaboration 65
Obstacles to Interdisciplinary Collaboration 67
Administrative Organization 67
Turf, Territory, and Competition 67
Differences in Professional Cultures 68
Professional Roles and Boundaries 69
Enhancing Interdisciplinary Collaboration 70
Commitment to Interdisciplinary Cooperation 70
Collaborative Program Development 71
Building Support for Interdisciplinary Collaboration 71
Managing Problems That Arise in Interdisciplinary Collaboration 72
Future Needs 72

Chapter 6. Collaboration in Programs for Children with Chronic Health Conditions and Their Families 75

Barriers to Collaborative Comprehensive Care 75
Developing Models of Collaborative Comprehensive Care 77
Collaborative Team Functioning 78
Tensions and Stresses in Collaborative Care 79
Collaborative Management of Chronic Psychophysiological Problems 80
Obstacles to Collaborative Management 81
Collaborative Management of Chronic Psychophysiological Problems 82
Program Development 82
Clinical Services: Example from the Program at CHOP 83
Research 85
Future Needs 86

Chapter 7. Research-Related Collaboration ... 89

Advantages of Collaborative Research ... 89
Models of Research-Related Collaboration ... 91
Facilitating Research-Related Collaboration ... 93
  Securing Time and Resources ... 93
  Developing Support for Collaborative Research ... 94
  Starting Small and Ending Up Big ... 95
Problematic Issues in Research-Related Collaboration ... 96
Future Directions ... 98
  Training for Collaborative Research ... 98
  Using Research to Develop New Clinical Programs ... 99
  Using Research to Develop Pediatric Psychology Programs ... 100

Chapter 8. Developing Pediatric Psychology Programs in Academic Medical Settings ... 101

Obstacles to Programmatic Collaboration ... 101
  Problematic Communication ... 101
  Problems in Administrative Organization ... 102
  Lack of Resources ... 103
  Conflicts among Psychologists ... 104
Ingredients of Successful Programmatic Collaboration ... 104
  Departmental Recognition of Psychologists' Contributions ... 105
  Clarity of Administrative Communication and Decision Making ... 106
  Leadership and Power ... 106
  Teamwork and Group Support ... 107
  Developing Economic Resources ... 107
  Examples of Program Development in Academic Medical Settings ... 107
Common Themes in Program Development ... 113
  Diversity of Funding Sources and Activities ... 113
  Core Administrative Identity as Psychologists ... 114
  Energetic, Supportive Leadership ... 114
Future Directions ... 114

Chapter 9. Professional and Ethical Issues in Collaboration ... 117

Confidentiality ... 117
Professional Boundaries in Patient Care ... 119
Conflict in Professional Roles ... 119

Interprofessional Tensions and Conflicts in Clinical Management 120
Conflicts in Expectations about Professional Roles 121
Addressing and Preventing Collaborative Conflicts 123
Practicing within Boundaries of Professional Competence 124
Long-Term Strategies to Enhance Professional Competence 125
Developing and Maintaining Professional Autonomy 126
Future Directions 127

Chapter 10. Empirical Studies of Consultation and Collaboration 129

Description of Psychological Consultation Services 129
Physicians' Utilization of Psychological Services 130
Pediatric Screening and Identification of Behavioral and Developmental Disorders 131
Pediatric Management of Specific Clinical Problems 132
Physicians' Perceptions of Psychological Services 134
Physicians' Satisfaction with Psychological Services 135
Physicians' Satisfaction with Psychological Consultation in Specific Settings 136
Acceptability of Psychological Services 137
Evaluation of Psychological Services in Primary Care Settings ... 138
Future Directions 141

Chapter 11. Training Psychologists in Consultation and Collaboration 143

Facilitating a Context for Teaching Collaboration 144
Training in Inpatient Consultation 145
Supervised Observations of Hopsital Rounds 145
Observations of Informal Contacts 145
Clinical Supervision 146
Training for Consultation in Primary Care 146
Common Dilemmas for Student Trainees 148
Training for Collaborative Research 150
Exposure to Models of Pediatric Practitioners and Researchers 150
Didactic Training 150
Collaborative Mentorship and Research Teams 151
Facilitating Student Research through Collaboration 152
Training and Support for Faculty 153
Support for Collaborative Teaching at a Regional Level 153
Future Directions 155

Part II: New Opportunities for Collaboration with Physicians

Introduction 157

Chapter 12. Developing a Collaborative Pediatric Psychology Practice in a Pediatric Primary Care Setting 159

Linda K. Hurley

Setting Up a Practice 160
Clinic Location and Structure 160
Negotiating with a Pediatric Group 161
Pediatric Psychology Practice Structure: Legal and Accounting Issues 162
Developing the Practice 164
Services 164
Reimbursement and Expenses 164
Marketing 165
Research 166
Developing Referrals 166
Parents' Perception of the Practice 167
Outside Contracts 168
Issues and Challenges 169
Ongoing Communication 169
Expanding the Practice 170
Implications for Training in Collaborative Practice 170
Managing the Future Challenges of Practice 171

Chapter 13. Collaborative Psychological Practice in Pediatric Gastroenterology: Clinical Issues and Professional Opportunities 173

Carin Cunningham

A Collaborative Practice Model 174
Evolution of the Practice 174
Description of the Practice 174
Summary of Clinical Services 175
Psychological Consultation for Specific Medical Problems 175
Inflammatory Bowel Disease 176
Encopresis 177
Ulcer Disease 177
Recurrent Abdominal Pain 177

Colitis 177
Feeding Problems 178
Collaborative Practice Issues 178
Management of Referrals and Communication 179
Case Examples of Clinical Consultation 179
Benefits of Collaborative Practice 181
Facilitating the Engagement of Children and Families in Assessment and Intervention 181
Mutual Learning 181
Problems in Collaborative Work 182
Integrating New Services into the Practice 182
Future Implications 184

Chapter 14. Consultation in an Adolescent Medicine Clinic .. 185

Susan L. Rosenthal

Need for Psychological Services in Adolescent Medicine 185
Consultation Issues in an Adolescent Clinic 186
Background Information Concerning the Clinic 186
Training 188
Training Psychologists 189
Enhancing Physicians' Knowledge of Adolescent Development 190
Clinical Care 191
Research 192
Collaborative Issues and Problems 192
Future Directions 193

Chapter 15. Psychological Consultation in Family Medicine .. 195

Peggy Crawford

Description of Setting 196
Types of Activities Conducted by Psychologists 196
Clinical Services and Teaching 197
Formal Teaching Activities 197
Obstacles to Collaboration 202

Chapter 16. New Opportunities for Collaboration: Implications 205

Developing Collaborative Relationships 205
Challenges of Integrating Psychology into Medical Settings 206
"It's Never Easy": Managing Collaborative Tensions 207

Chapter 17. Anticipating the Future of Collaboration 209

Pediatric Work Force Trends and Practice Patterns 209
Challenges to Collaboration 210
Impact of Health Care Reform 212
Strategies to Enhance Future Collaborative Efforts 214
Specialization 214
Collaborative Clinical Management 214
Collaborative Training Activities 215
Collaborative Research Opportunities 215
Collaboration between AAP and APA 216
Task Force on Coding for Mental Health in Children 216
Collaborative Advocacy in Service Development and Policy ... 217
Facilitating Program and Professional Development 219

Epilogue: Reflections on Lessons Learned in Collaboration 221

What Can Psychologists Learn from Pediatricians? 221
Clinical Experience and Perspective 221
Advocacy 222
Enhancing the Practical Application of Psychological Research 222
What Makes an Effective Psychological Consultant? 222
Training and Experience 223
Personal Attributes 223
Sustaining Consultation and Collaboration over Time 224
Setting Realistic Expectations 224
Diversity of Activities 225
Flexibility in Managing Change 225

References 227

Index 241

Introduction

One hallmark of pediatric psychology is the interaction and communication with pediatricians and other physicians. Such collaboration takes many forms and requires a wide range of skills. Consider the following example. A pediatrician, Dr. X, contacts a psychologist to discuss an 8-year-old child whose symptoms of abdominal pain have been associated with frequent school absence. Dr. X reports that this level of school absence is unusual and that the child's symptoms do not correspond to the negative findings of a medical exam. Dr. X makes the following request: "I'm not sure where to go from here; can you take a look at this child and let me know what you think? By the way, the parents are convinced that Sam's problems relate to organic disease, even though I've reassured them that I don't think this is the case. I'm not sure they will contact you."

It turns out that Sam's parents do contact the psychologist, whose assessment reveals that Sam is very worried about leaving his mother to attend school partly because he is concerned about his mother's health. His mother has had a history of cancer, and the entire family has been worried about a recurrence. The psychologist informs Dr. X of these findings, and together they decide on a collaborative plan that includes a referral of Sam's mother to her physician for a reexamination, ongoing pediatric monitoring of Sam's symptoms, and psychological intervention. The psychologist initiates a discussion and clarification of the family's fears about Sam's physical health and that of his mother and develops a family plan to structure and support Sam's school attendance. After several months, the psychologist and Dr. X discuss Sam's progress by phone. He is now attending school more regularly, and his symptoms have lessened. In this case example, what look like straightforward, routine characteristics of consultation concerning patient care actually reflect some complex questions such as the following. What about this child's problem reached the threshold to trigger Dr. X's referral to a psychologist? How did the physician choose this particular psychologist? What did the psychologist say to Dr. X in giving feedback about the referral? How did they coordinate their contacts with Sam's family?

Collaborations with pediatricians are not restricted to individual cases such as Sam's but occur at many levels that influence the development of the field of pediatric psychology as well as the professional development and opportunities of individual psychologists. Consider the following example: Faculty pediatricians in a growing department of pediatrics have been interested for some time in expanding the level of available mental health services for children at their hospital. Individually, they have had some experience with various mental health professionals, including psychologists. However, as a faculty they are not sure which direction to take in developing their program. As they begin to discuss their experiences and opinions, several questions arise. What specific contributions can a psychologist make to services at their hospital and to the growth of their department? How do psychologists' skills and experience differ from those of other professionals? Do psychologists have sufficient experience with medical patients to manage complex cases? Will the residents accept teaching from a psychologist? How much of a psychologist's salary can be recovered through insurance and fee for services? The answers to such questions, which are clearly important to physicians and hospital administrators in many settings, depend heavily on the quality of their experiences in working with individual psychologists.

In the course of their practice, research, teaching, and administrative efforts, psychologists and pediatricians communicate and collaborate in many different ways and in many settings. To ensure continued development of the field of pediatric psychology, one can anticipate that future practice, research, and training will necessitate even closer interdisciplinary communication and collaboration in an ever-widening range of settings. Consequently, pediatric psychologists and their physician colleagues will need to consider several difficult questions that are involved in interdisciplinary consultation and collaboration. What are the essential ingredients of effective consultation and collaboration? How can consultation and collaboration be made more effective and efficient? What are the most salient obstacles to interprofessional collaboration? What training is necessary to enhance the level and quality of consultation and collaboration among psychologists and pediatricians? Beyond working in individual patient care situations, what can be done to enhance frequency and quality of collaboration among psychologists and pediatricians to develop service programs, research, and advocacy to enhance the lives of children and their families?

To address these and other related questions, this volume is organized around critical issues concerning the content of collaborative activities and the settings in which these activities take place. The book begins with an introduction and historical overview of the roots of interdisciplinary collaboration and implications for current practice. Chapter 2 presents a descriptive model of.collaborative activities and influences. The next two chapters concern collaborative work and consultation in primary care and inpatient settings. Subsequent chapters are devoted to relevant content areas such as collaborating with other professions, collaboration in programs for children with chronic health conditions, collaborative research, professional and ethical issues, programmatic collaboration, empirical evaluation, and training.

The next section of the book brings together several psychologists who report their recent experiences in areas that have not been well described but are likely to be "hot" areas of future collaboration. These include starting a collaborative pediatric psychology practice, experiences in a collaborative practice with pediatric gastroenterology, consultation in an adolescent medicine clinic, and consultation in family medicine. The book concludes with a chapter that anticipates future directions and an epilogue that summarizes final reflections.

CONSULTING WITH PHYSICIANS OTHER THAN PEDIATRICIANS

An increasing number of psychologists work and consult with medical practitioners (e.g., family practice and adolescent medicine specialists, etc.) other than pediatricians. Moreover, some pediatric subspecialists identify themselves primarily as subspecialists, e.g., as oncologists rather than as pediatricians. One of the dilemmas I had in writing this book was to try to reconcile my interest in considering consultation with a broad range of medical practitioners with the need to write from my own experience, which primarily involves pediatricians and pediatric subspecialists. The title of the book and the focus of most chapters reflect my experience with pediatric colleagues. However, readers should understand that many of the issues in consultation and collaboration that are covered in this book are generalizable beyond pediatricians. For example, the description of models of collaborative activities and influences that is presented in Chapter 2 is applicable to consultation with other physicians. Moreover, my recognition of the importance of psychologists' collaborative activities with a range of physicians also led me to invite chapters (Chapters 13–15) that deal specifically with psychological consultation in adolescent medicine, family practice, and gastroenterology. Interested readers can obtain a feel for the similarities and differences in consultation with different medical practitioners by considering this material. Moreover, readers who consult with physicians other than pediatricians concerning children's problems might want to substitute "physician" for "pediatrician" as they read this book.

Part I

1

Evolution of Collaboration among Psychologists and Pediatricians

A Brief History

The professions of psychology and medicine have had separate origins, and each has undergone major transformations in the 20th century (Starr, 1982; Routh, 1994; Sarason, 1981). Based on these descriptions, I think it is safe to say that both groups have spent most of their energies in extending their own influence, resolving various professional/developmental crises, and in specialization rather than in interprofessional cooperation. However, even a brief history uncovers some interesting roots of interprofessional collaboration that have clear implications for modern efforts. These developments are reviewed in this chapter.

DEVELOPMENT OF PEDIATRICS IN THE UNITED STATES

Pediatrics is itself a relatively recent medical specialty, and developmental and behavioral pediatrics are even newer. From its origins, a continuing theme of the specialty of pediatrics has been involvement with social movements promoting the welfare of children (Abt, 1965; Halpern, 1988; Harvey, 1993). The earliest pediatricians who practiced in the latter half of the century were practitioners of general medicine who built part-time practices in newly established institutions for abandoned and destitute children, orphanages, foundling homes, and dispensaries (Halpern, 1988). Clinical experiences with pediatric problems, the emergence of training centers and children's hospitals, and the individual careers of early pediatric pioneers formed the foundation for specialty of pediatrics. For example, Abraham Jacobi, recognized as one of the first American physicians to devote himself to the care of children, was appointed Professor of Infantile Pathology and Therapeutics at New York Medical College and started the first pediatric clinic in the United States (Harvey, 1993). The emergency of specialized professional practice was reflected in the founding of the Section on Diseases of Children (1880) and the American Pediatric Society (1899) and in publications including *Archives of Pediatrics* (1884), *Pediatrics* (1896), and Holt's *Diseases of Infancy and Childhood* (1896), which is recognized as the pediatric text in longest continuous circulation (Harvey, 1993).

The central problems that preoccupied early pediatricians in what Richmond (1967) has described as the prescientific era of pediatrics were infection, nutrition, infant formula preparation, and high infant mortality. In the early 1900s, pediatricians focused a great deal on the study and dissemination of feeding information to help prevent the problems associated with malnutrition among economically disadvantaged infants. Unfortunately, such problems are still very much with us today and still require collaborative solutions (Frank & Drotar, 1994). The development of the profession and practice of pediatrics was facilitated by federal legislation such as the creation of the Children's Bureau in 1913 to study and monitor infant mortality. In the early 1900s, infant welfare clinics and urban health centers established through the Sheppard–Towner Act of 1921, the first Federal program for mothers and children, provided funds for states to provide disadvantaged mothers and children with prenatal care, health supervision, and advice concerning infant feeding.

The founding of the American Academy of Pediatrics (AAP) in 1930 was clearly an important milestone in the history of pediatrics in this country. Interestingly, one impetus for the formation of the Academy was a conflict with the American Medical Association (AMA) concerning the Sheppard–Towner Act. According to Hughes (1993), the AMA was strongly opposed to this legislation, regarding it as socialistic government interference, and even reprimanded the member Section on Pediatrics for its approval of the law. However, convinced that such legislation was in the best interests of mothers and children, the Section refused to recant. Pediatricians eventually recognized that the AMA was not the primary organization through which they could work to improve the health and welfare of children. A strong emphasis on promoting public policy to improve the lives of children and their families and their access to health care continues in the current agenda of the AAP (*AAP Status Report on Initiatives*, February, 1993a).

By the 1930s, the scope of pediatric practice broadened with the development of the well-baby conference, which involved frequent periodic medical consultation and increasing focus on physical growth and child development (Halpern, 1988). Such practice paved the way for modern-day collaboration as exemplified in Gesell's (1926) plea for psychological norms "to lay down for various ages of infancy and childhood certain concrete minimum essentials of normal health expressed in tangible behavior terms" (p. 48). Other forerunners of modern-day behavioral pediatricians such as Fife (1934) described the pediatrician's responsibility "to search out early manifestations of biologic instability and behavioral problems" (p. 19).

On the other hand, some early pediatricians were downright suspicious of collaboration with other professions. In a provocative paper, "Pediatric Psychology and the Child Guidance Movement," Brenneman (1932) warned about the potential negative effects of the child guidance movement. In his discussion, psychiatrists and psychologists were lumped together as "child guiders" and said to cause parents needless worries about their child's feeding behavior and psychological development.

EARLY DEVELOPMENTS IN COLLABORATION

Between the problems of malnourished children seen in ambulatory pediatric care and the children in foundling homes and hospitals, there would have been plenty of work for pediatric psychologists, had this specialty existed in the early and mid-1900s. Surprisingly, there were a few psychologist practitioners in pediatric settings even then. Routh (1994) cited the work of Jean W. McFarlane, who later went on to a distinguished career in child development, who practiced as a psychologist at a children's hospital in San Francisco as early as 1917–1918. There may have been others, but written records are hard to come by.

Although strong interests in interdisciplinary efforts were by no means typical for pediatricians and psychologists, past or present, several early visionaries had marked collaborative predilections that exemplified contrasting models of interprofessional relationships (Routh, 1990). Such pioneers included individual practitioners such as the psychologist Lightmer Witmer, who had interests in psychology and pediatrics, Arnold Gesell, who combined the two disciplines of pediatrics and psychology in a "single skull" (Routh, 1990), and pediatric researchers such as John Anderson and Milton Senn, who had strong interests in child psychology.

The founder of the first psychological clinic in 1899, Lightmer Witmer, was on the editorial board of a pediatric journal and consulted with pediatricians (Routh, 1990; Peterson & Harbeck, 1988). However, the nature and depth of Witmer's collaborative relationships with pediatricians are not clear from published work. Arnold Gesell, stands out as a highly unusual figure whose career bridged pediatrics and psychology. A forerunner of modern-day developmental and behavioral pediatricians, Gesell complemented his Ph.D. in psychology with an M.D. and was among the first to discuss the need for clinical psychologists to manage psychological problems of children in medical settings (Gesell, 1919). He was also instrumental in founding and directing the Yale Clinic for Child Development, which had a long tradition of interdisciplinary research and clinical service.

Probably because relatively few psychologists were practicing, the first descriptions of collaborative possibilities were written by pediatricians. In an interesting paper of some historical significance, Anderson (1930) was among the first to describe potential contributions of psychology to pediatrics such as developmental research and the role of intelligence testing as a means of understanding individual variation among children. In his presidential address to the American Pediatric Society, Wilson (1964) exhorted practicing pediatricians to employ their own clinical psychologists as a means of helping to manage the emotional and behavioral problems of children, thus presaging many developments in modern collaborative practice.

As described by Senn (1975), research in child development provided the most solid collaborative bridge among many professions, including psychologists and pediatricians, during the early to mid-1900s. Stimulated by funds from the Laura Spelman Rockefeller Memorial Fund, several universities established interdisciplinary child development institutes that conducted research on various aspects of physical and psychological development. In the 1920s and 1930s, several child development research programs, e.g., Fels Research Institute, Yale Child Study Center, were established under the direction of physicians. The founding of the Society for Research in Child Development (SRCD) in 1930 was a related and very critical development (Anderson, 1956). To this day, SRCD is an primary example of an organization that has helped to establish and promote interdisciplinary research and policy efforts. Developmental psychologists and pediatricians have served as presidents and officers of this organization.

Among the researchers of this time, Milton Senn, a pediatrician, was noteworthy for his promotion of collaboration among many professors, including pediatric and developmental psychology, at the Institute of Child Development in the Department of Pediatrics at the New York Hospital–Cornell Medical Center and subsequently at Yale Child Study Center. Senn's (1975) personal reflections about interdisciplinary work in this setting presage the collaborative dilemmas of modern times: "On paper the Yale set-up was ideal, but in actuality the relationships between the Child Study Center and the various departments were often strained . . . problems of territorial rights, competition between departments and the struggle for funds impeded the effort" (p. 61). Does any of this sound familiar?

Coincident with such pioneering research collaborations, the profession of pediatrics was undergoing what Levine (1950) described as its golden age of curative pediatrics, which included "prophylactic immunization, widespread use of vitamins, nutritional knowledge, water and electrolyte metabolism, discovery and availability of antibiotics, isolation and synthesis of hormones" (p. 651). Subsequent to 1950 and continuing into the present, pediatrics entered an age of specialization. Board certification, which was established first in cardiology in 1960, is now available in a large number of specialties, with more anticipated. Such specialization has continuing implications for the nature of collaboration with psychologists.

THE EMERGENCE OF DEVELOPMENTAL AND BEHAVIORAL PEDIATRICS

According to Halpern (1988), various forces, such as a drop in the birth rate leading to unfavorable market conditions, tensions in subspecialized training versus general pediatrics, and the necessity to increase the status and scientific basis of pediatrics, eventually resulted in a movement to integrate child development and behavior into pediatric training and practice. This call to arms was championed by a group of pediatric leaders whose writings and professional influence have helped to shape modern-day behavioral and developmental pediatrics, including prospects for interdisciplinary collaboration. For example, in his influential address, "Child Development as a Basic Science for Pediatrics," Richmond (1967) recognized that the field of pediatrics had entered an era of child development and prevention. In Richmond's view, the future of pediatrics called for a strategy for incorporating teaching and research in child development into the mainstream of pediatrics, including the development of "a core of pediatric faculty members with a disciplined background of research and teaching analogous to our academic colleagues in metabolism, infectious disease, etc." (p. 141). Richmond also highlighted the relevance of child development, psychology, and other sciences for the practice of pediatrics.

Another well-respected, highly influential pediatric leader, Robert Haggerty, has consistently championed interdisciplinary research and practice through his writings, mentorship, and leadership of the William T.

Grant Foundation. Like Richmond, Haggerty recognized and appreciated the significance of changes in the practice of pediatrics. In a very influential book, Haggerty, Roghmann, and Pless (1975) noted:

> a group of new childhood difficulties that we have termed the "new morbidity" is now gaining attention. Many of these difficulties lie beyond the boundaries of traditional medical care. The most prominent of the child health problems that have emerged in the past decade or two are behavioral and school problems found in children of all ages . . . Underlying some of the new morbidity are problems arising from modern society such as social and geographic mobility, crowding, high rise living and urban decay. Other problems (alcohol, drugs, venereal disease) are old, but their diffusion to younger and younger age groups and lessening of social contacts make them concerns for pediatricians and parents (pp. 94–95)

One salient consequence of the "new morbidity" was the requirement for greater collaboration with other health professionals, including psychologists (Haggerty, 1986). As director of the William T. Grant Foundation from 1980 to 1992, Haggerty sponsored the development of interdisciplinary research consortia that would bring together scientists from a broad range of disciplines, including pediatricians and psychologists, to combine their efforts to enhance scientific progress in various fields, e.g., chronic illness in children, divorce and children, and ethnicity and adolescent development.

As these pediatric leaders and others such as Green (1985) began to describe and define the field of behavioral and developmental pediatrics, deficiencies in pediatricians' training in these areas of practice became more apparent (Task Force on Pediatric Education, 1978). To address these needs, pediatricians have involved psychologists and others in pediatric training, which has become one major focus of collaboration (Davidson, 1988).

Specialized professional identities of a new breed of pediatricians were reflected in the formation of the Society for Developmental Pediatrics (SDP) in 1978 and the Society for Behavioral Pediatrics (SBP) in 1982. From its inception the SBP has been an interdisciplinary organization that has very much welcomed the participation of psychologists and other professions. Psychologists are well represented on the editorial board of the *Journal of Developmental and Behavioral Pediatrics* and hold office on the Executive Council of SBP. Moreover, the Society of Pediatric Psychology (SPP) maintains an active liaison with the SBP. The first National Conference on Behavioral Pediatrics, which was held in Easton, Maryland in 1985 (Wender & Friedman, 1985), helped to define this emerging field with descriptions of teaching and clinical roles (Green, 1985) and interdisciplinary collaboration (Drotar, 1985; Friedman, 1985).

DEVELOPMENTS IN PEDIATRICIAN/PSYCHOLOGIST COLLABORATION

The above developments in the profession of pediatrics certainly created a climate that was hospitable to those pioneering psychologists who gradually entered collaborative waters in clinical service, training, and research.

Early Clinical Collaborations

To my knowledge, two pediatricians, Smith and Rome, and a psychologist, Freedheim (1967), reported the first general and data-based description of collaborative clinical practice, which is the forerunner of the conjoint-practice model of today (Schroeder & Mann, 1991). According to these authors, advantages of this half-day-a-week practice model included parental preferences for the psychologist within the office, improved access, and reduction of parents' resistance to referral, giving children and families the opportunity to observe the "natural relationship between the psychologist and the pediatrician availability of the complete medical records and communication" (p. 48). The authors held monthly meetings to discuss cases and share mutual learning experiences and provide direct service evaluation and short-term interventions including behavioral management, e.g., discipline, toileting, school-related problems, adolescent adjustment, adjustment to divorce, and mental retardation. The majority of children (61%) were seen for three visits or fewer (Smith, Rome, & Freedheim, 1967). D. K. Freedheim (personal communication, Nov. 5, 1993) noted that this practice arrangement continued for several years but then evolved into an interdependent practice of pediatric psychology as other community pediatricians began to refer their patients.

Early Collaborative Teaching and Training Efforts

As noted by Routh (1975), one of the earliest efforts in collaborative teaching was a committee on the relations between psychology and medical education that was established by the American Psychological Association in 1911 (Fernberger, 1932). The early growth of psychologists in medical schools was relatively slow. In the early 1940s, fewer than a dozen medical schools had a psychologist on the faculty (Mensh, 1953). In keeping with the rapid growth of clinical psychology in schools of medicine, the number of psychologists in medical school departments, including pediatrics, increased significantly in the post-World War II era, presumably as a response to available resources and interest in expanding teaching programs. By 1955, Matarazzo and Daniel (1957) reported that medical school faculties listed an average of over four psychologists.

As is true today, psychologists in these early teaching programs were much more involved in teaching pediatricians than pediatricians were in training psychologists. One notable exception was the first pediatric psychology graduate training program at the University of Iowa (Routh, 1969). The brainchild of Gerald Solomons, a developmental pediatrician, and Leonard Eron, a psychologist, both of whom have had distinguished careers in their respective fields, this NIH-supported training program was designed partly to train pediatricians in child development by requiring them to seek a Ph.D. in child development. This program did not identify any pediatricians who wanted this training. However, the program facilitated the careers of psychologists, including this author, by involving them in clinical training in an interdisciplinary clinical practice setting, a child development clinic at the University of Iowa Hospital school, and course work in child development coupled with rigorous research training, Iowa style. Although I did not realize it at the time, this program would have an extraordinary influence on my professional development by giving me a first-hand opportunity to observe competent pediatric and psychologist clinicians and researchers in cooperative work. Starting with my first year of graduate school and continuing throughout my graduate training, I observed and received feedback from pediatricians, speech pathologists, and educational specialists, among others, and learned to place a high priority on interdisciplinary research and practice.

Training activities also proved to be an important collaborative inroad for psychologists in medical school settings. By 1970, Routh's landmark survey of each of the 100 U.S. medical school departments found that the majority (61) had at least one psychologist affiliated with their department. A substantial number (more than half) participated in some kind of training of psychologists. These programs and the types of collaboration they reflect were as diverse as they are today and include developmental psychology research and research training ($n = 8$); clinical psychology (practicum, internship, postdoctoral) ($n = 41$); developmental clinical programs combining service and research ($n = 7$); and programs involving training of pediatricians in developmental or clinical psychology ($n = 14$) (Routh, 1970).

Routh (1972) repeated the survey to determine whether pediatric psychology was capable of surviving the harsher professional climate of the 1970s, e.g., cutbacks in training and government funds and a gloomy job market, factors that sound remarkably similar to the 1990s. On the basis of the increased number of pediatric departments with some kind of psychological training activity and increases in the number and variety of developmental clinical psychology activities, especially multidisciplinary clinics for management of developmental disorders, Routh (1972) concluded that developmental psychology was holding its own and that clinical psychology was flourishing in departments of pediatrics. It would be instructive to repeat this survey today.

EARLY VISIONS OF COLLABORATION: PSYCHOLOGISTS' VIEWS

The first psychologist to report a published vision of psychologist–pediatrician collaboration was the renowned developmental psychologist Jerome Kagan, whose address on the occasion of the opening of the renovated pediatric clinic at the Massachusetts General Hospital in Boston was published in 1965 in the *American Journal of Diseases of Children*. Kagan's vision of the relationship between psychology and pediatrics was bold: he proposed nothing less than a marriage. Psychologists would have the benefit of direct observation with psychopathology and developmental problems; pediatricians would have the opportunity to think theoretically about the etiology of symptoms and to become acquainted with research inquiry. Kagan's description of the empirical and clinical products of this marriage included the following: (1) relationships of prenatal and perinatal factors to psychological problems; (2) early detection of severe childhood disturbances, especially schizophrenia; (3) early detection of psychosocial problems, e.g., academic retardation, delinquency, psychosomatic disturbances, and phobias; and (4) application of theory and research to therapy with psychological problems. Kagan was prophetic. Pediatricians and psychologists have engaged in collaborative practice and research on all of these topics, though much remains to be accomplished.

Wright's widely cited (1967) description of the roles of the pediatric psychologist embraced Kagan's metaphor of the marriage between pediatrics and psychology and looked forward to such "blessed events" as psychological pediatricians, described as scholar professionals trained both as physicians and behavioral scientists (who certainly resemble today's behavioral and developmental pediatricians), and pediatric psychologists trained in child development and child clinical psychology. In order to achieve optimal collaboration with their pediatric colleagues, Wright (1967) urged psychologists to thoroughly understand the requirements of pediatric practice and to develop and utilize assessment methods and brief, prevention-focused treatments that fit best with this setting. Like

Kagan, Wright (1967) foretold the future in his description of three professional trends including (1) clear delineation of the role of the pediatric psychologist, (2) more specific training for personnel who plan to enter this area, and (3) construction of a new body of knowledge.

On the other hand, it should be noted that not every psychologist embraced the metaphor of the marriage between psychology and pediatrics. For example, Cushna (1968) expressed concern that expecting a blessed event between psychologists and pediatricians might produce "immature interspecies mules" (p. 288). In their description of psychological training in a pediatric practice, Fisher and Engeln (1972) described remarkably modern collaborative problems such as difficulty in the setting of fees and securing sufficient space for the psychologist's clinical work. Following Kagan and Wright, one of the first to describe the practical applications of the pediatric psychologist's collaborative activities was Salk (1970), who articulated a role for psychologists in "on the spot consultation" (p. 395) that clearly fit with pediatricians' action-oriented approach. Salk's model is quite modern in that it features close integration of the psychologist's work with that of the pediatrician in immediate discussion of the case, screening, early diagnosis, and/or appointment for psychological services. This "pediatrician-friendly" consultation model was a powerful influence on one of Salk's students, Gail Gardner, who was the first editor of the *Pediatric Psychology Newsletter* and an influential clinical mentor in my career.

MODERN GROWTH OF COLLABORATION

The frequency and depth of grass roots collaboration grew in response to developments in service, teaching, and research made by pediatricians and psychologists with interests in pediatric populations. The formation of the Society of Pediatric Psychology (SPP) in 1968, which had grown to 650 members by 1972, provided a professional affiliation and "home" for psychologists in pediatric settings. Not surprisingly, issues related to collaboration were among the major concerns expressed by pediatric psychologists in published writings (Ack, 1974; Botinelli, 1975; Schroeder, Goolsby, & Stangler, 1974). Special issues of the *Journal of Clinical Child Psychology*, including Volume 4 (No. 3), 1975, "Pediatric Psychology," and Volume 7 (No. 6), 1978, "Clinical Child Psychologists and Primary Health Care Providers," advanced the field by describing a rich mix of collaborative and consultative efforts. Psychologists' interests in interdisciplinary collaboration in health care settings became profession-wide as evidenced by a special issue of *Professional Psychology* (Volume 10, No. 4,

1979) that was devoted entirely to psychologists in health care settings. In 1982, the April issue of the *Pediatric Clinics of North America* (Volume 29, No. 2) focused on behavioral pediatrics. This volume featured discussions by pediatric leaders, e.g., Haggerty (1982) and Chamberlin (1982), on such topics as prevention and early identification of behavioral disorders, and by psychologists such as Christophersen (1982), who described how behavioral approaches could be incorporated into pediatric practice.

The interdisciplinary efforts that began with the Easton conference (Wender & Friedman, 1985) have continued up to the present time in various forms. For example, in 1989, the National Institutes of Child Health and Human Development and the Maternal and Child Health Research Branch of the Bureau of Health Care Delivery and Assistance jointly sponsored a conference, Research in Behavioral Pediatrics, in Columbia, Maryland. Primary conference goals were to identify directions for future research and to enhance interdisciplinary collaborative research efforts within the field of behavioral pediatrics. Toward this end, psychologists and pediatricians collaborated on state-of-the-art papers concerning various topics (e.g., injury, childhood asthma) as models of research (see *Pediatrics*, 90, 1992, Supplement). Interdisciplinary collaboration figured prominently in discussions of the future of behavioral pediatrics research (Green, Boyle, Finney, Phillips, & Zuckerman, 1992).

Finally, collaboration and consultation have clearly emerged as a consistent theme in the writings of influential pediatric psychologists (Roberts & Wright, 1982; Stabler, 1988; Stabler & Mesibov, 1984; Tuma, 1982). The cumulative force of this work presages a healthy future for cooperative work among pediatricians and psychologists. However, that is getting ahead of the story. First, I need to tell you about the present state of collaborative work between these professions.

2

Models of Collaborative Activities and Influences

Interdisciplinary collaboration can be defined as a professional activity or interaction that is conducted between members of two professions (Drotar, 1993). Collaboration occurs among individuals, which is how we usually think of it, at a program level, i.e., among groups of psychologists and pediatricians in a particular setting, or among professional organizations (Wright, 1985). Although professional writings tend to focus on collaboration between individual practitioners, contextual or system influences are also important (Mullins, Gillman, & Harbeck, 1992).

Understanding of interprofessional collaboration has been limited by definitional and conceptual problems. Although collaborative work involves a broad spectrum of activities, the essential feature is the relationship among collaborators. Unfortunately, professional guidelines that concern the conduct of interprofessional relationships, including collaborative roles and responsibilities, are ambiguous. Moreover, the factors that influence these activities are not well understood (Drotar, 1993). To address this need, this chapter presents a descriptive framework for interdisciplinary models of collaboration and influences (Drotar, 1993).

DESCRIPTION OF COLLABORATIVE ACTIVITIES

As shown in Table 1, the primary characteristics of these activities encompass five dimensions: (1) the content or goal of the collaborative activity, (2) setting(s) in which these activities take place, (3) characteristics of participants, including prior experience in collaboration and current roles, (4) characteristics of the collaborative relationship, and (5) outcomes.

Table 1. Dimensions of Collaborative Activities among Psychologists and Pediatricians

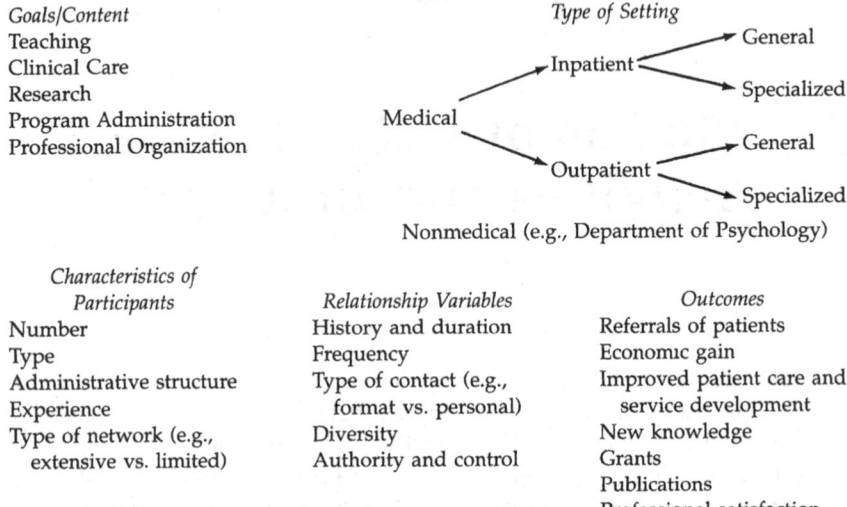

Goals/Content
- Teaching
- Clinical Care
- Research
- Program Administration
- Professional Organization

Type of Setting
- Medical
  - Inpatient
    - General
    - Specialized
  - Outpatient
    - General
    - Specialized
- Nonmedical (e.g., Department of Psychology)

Characteristics of Participants	*Relationship Variables*	*Outcomes*
Number	History and duration	Referrals of patients
Type	Frequency	Economic gain
Administrative structure	Type of contact (e.g., format vs. personal)	Improved patient care and service development
Experience	Diversity	New knowledge
Type of network (e.g., extensive vs. limited)	Authority and control	Grants
		Publications
		Professional satisfaction

From *Journal of Pediatric Psychology, Vol 18,* 1993, p. 162.

Goal or Content

The goals of collaboration include the familiar areas of patient care, teaching, and research as well as several others that are not as well recognized, such as program administration or collaboration between professional organizations such as the American Psychological Association (APA) and the American Academy of Pediatrics (AAP). Consultation is a subset of collaborative activities that focus on a specific problem, e.g., a pediatrician requests a psychologist's opinion concerning management of a child with a behavior problem. Several chapters in this book are organized around the primary goals of collaborative work, e.g., research, teaching, program development.

Settings

Collaborative activities between psychologists and pediatricians occur in diverse settings with populations and work-related demands that influence professional needs and expectations. These settings include primary care or inpatient hospital settings, which may be general or specialized, e.g., a unit for children with cancer. Of necessity, interdisciplinary collaboration should be tailored to specific settings. This specialized emphasis is reflected in chapters on consultation and collaboration in primary care, inpatient settings, and in the "new directions" section, which describes collaborative work in general and specialized pediatric practices, adolescent medicine, and family practice.

Characteristics of Collaborators

The nature of one's prior clinical experience, especially in interprofessional work, will often shape collaborative goals and expectations. For example, limited contact among potential collaborators could contribute to a stereotyped perception; e.g., psychologists are only good for testing. Psychologists who have not had much experience with pediatricians often underestimate the demands of pediatric practice and/or fail to address the practical relevance of their assessments or interventions to pediatric practice.

The nature and quality of prior collaborative experiences also affect colleagues' expectations. For example, successful collaborative experiences might be expected to lead to positive attitudes toward future collaboration and higher rates of requests for consultation, whereas negative experiences would dampen enthusiasm and lessen requests for future cooperative work. Consequently, successful collaborative programs are characterized by relatively high levels of satisfaction among colleagues and increasing requests for collaborative help.

Collaborators' current work expectations and demands also exert a powerful influence on their collaborative expectations. For example, pediatric house staff on an inpatient service must rapidly broker a great many consultation requests to different subspecialists and professions in a rapid time frame. For this reason they place a high value on the speed of the psychologist's response. In this context, even the most thorough or thoughtful psychological consultation is of little help if it is late. In contrast, although private pediatric practitioners also operate under considerable time constraints, their professional livelihoods are heavily dependent on the satisfaction of the consumers of their service. For this reason, one would expect them to place a high value on the psychologist's ability to relate positively to patients and their parents and to make a positive impact on the referring problem. One of the consistent themes of this book is the need for successful collaborators to be mindful of their colleagues' work-related demands and, where possible, to try to accommodate to them.

The extensiveness of one's collaborative network is another potential influence. Psychologists who work with only two or three other physicians in a group practice generally have greater opportunities to personally influence colleagues than their counterparts at teaching hospitals who interact with a very large number of physicians (Drotar, 1993). Consequently, effective collaboration tends to be specialized and focused on several colleagues rather than dispersed among a large cast of potential collaborators.

Outcomes

Collaborative activities generate outcomes or products that function as incentives or disincentives for future efforts. Familiar examples of tangible products include a written report to a pediatrician about a recommended management plan following a psychological assessment, publications or grants resulting from cooperative research, or new clinical services or research that result from programmatic collaboration. Participants' personal reactions to and perceptions of collaborative work, e.g., personal satisfaction and stimulation, are less tangible but nonetheless important incentives (Drotar, Sturm, Eckerle, & White, 1993a).

Relationship Characteristics and Outcome

The quality of the relationship that develops among colleagues, which is arguably a central characteristic of collaborative work, is perhaps the least well understood dimension. Potentially salient characteristics include the history and duration of a collaborative relationship, the frequency and diversity of interprofessional contacts as well as qualitative features, such as how control and authority are managed in the relationship, and satisfaction. Interprofessional relationships are complex in that they often involve formal professional roles as well as personal elements such as mutual disclosure and a sense of trust that develop from a shared history (Rogers & Holloway, 1993).

Stages of Collaborative Relationships

Stages of collaborative relationships also need to be considered. In the initial phase, decisions about whether to work together, whom to work with, and for what purpose are most critical. Time-limited collaborations that focus on a specific patient or research problem are typical of this initial phase. However, following their participation in successful and/or satisfying interactions, collaborating workers may enter a different phase that is no longer solely focused on a specific clinical problem but includes more extensive reciprocal problem solving, planning, or decision making (Stabler, 1988). By definition, as collaborative relationships become more extensive, they require greater personal commitment and investment of time and energy than in the initial phases (Drotar & Sturm, in press).

MODELS OF COLLABORATION/CONSULTATION IN PEDIATRIC PSYCHOLOGY

Pediatric psychologists have described a range of collaborative models that focus mostly on clinical consultation in patient care or teaching. These models have been influenced by Caplan (1970), who distinguished among several different types of consultation such as client-centered, where the primary goal for the consultant is to develop a plan to help a client who has been referred by another professional, consultee-centered, where the primary focus is placed on increasing a professional's understanding and/or emotional mastery of issues involved in caring for a client or patient, and administrative consultation. Roberts and Wright (1982) have described three basic models of psychological consultation in pediatric settings: (1) independent functions; (2) indirect consultation; and (3) collaborative team models (see also Stabler, 1979). A fourth model, the systems-based approach (Mullins *et al.*, 1992), also merits consideration. The advantages and disadvantages of these models will now be considered.

Independent Functions Model

The independent functions model is most familiar to the pediatrician because it is very similar to medical consultation (Freidson, 1970). In this model, the psychologist functions as a specialist who provides diagnosis and, in some instances, treatment of a patient referred by the pediatrician. Collaboration primarily takes the form of information exchange prior to and after the referral. One advantage of this model ironically stems from the relatively low level of contact between the pediatrician and the psychologist and the limited time required. A second major advantage is the pediatrician's familiarity and comfort with this model. All pediatricians have had experience in arranging for consultation with other medical subspecialists during their training and later in practice and are familiar with the professional roles involved. Finally, this model is efficient, reasonably cost effective, and useful to the pediatrician and family.

The main disadvantages of this model of consultation involve the limited communication and relationships between professions. Pediatricians may structure the psychologist's consultation role incorrectly or too narrowly (Stabler & Murray, 1973). Moreover, the lack of opportunity for extensive dialogue between the pediatrician and the psychologist limits teaching opportunities and discussion of management alternatives. Stabler (1988) has described some excellent examples of such problems. Certain clinical problems, especially those that involve complex psychophysiological problems such as failure to thrive, require a high level of interdisciplinary communication that often cannot be effectively or exclusively managed within an independent functions model.

Indirect Consultation Model

An alternative approach is the indirect psychological consultation or process–educative model (Stabler, 1979). The hallmark of this model is that the pediatrician retains sole responsibility for clinical management while the psychologist assumes the role of teacher or informed colleague who provides advice, teaching, or protocols for patient management (Roberts, 1986).

Depending on the clinical problem, nature of collaborative relationship, or setting, the process–educative consultation model may take many forms. The informal hallway consultation is a time-honored method. For example, a pediatrician happens to see a psychologist lurking in the hall and asks her for advice about a troublesome patient. Such requests may be couched in many forms and guises, e.g., "What would you think of a 3-year-old boy who isn't talking?" "I have a family that is driving me crazy;" "I just received this report from the school psychologist, and I can't make heads or tails of it;" "What do you do for a child who refuses to go to school?" "How do I get treatment for this child? He seems depressed." Roberts (1986) noted that common questions for the indirect model include (1) whether a particular child's behavior is appropriate for age and possible intervention, (2) interpretation of psychological test data, (3) availability of community services for children with particular problems, and (4) need or appropriateness of a referral for psychological services. Such informal interchanges present useful potential opportunities for teaching, especially for sharpening referral questions, educating pediatricians concerning what a psychological evaluation can and cannot contribute, how best to present the need for a psychological evaluation to a family. However, this can be a very demanding and time-consuming method of teaching. It is difficult to generate clinical pearls rapidly or calmly when one is on the way to see a patient, teach a conference, or on the way to the bathroom, or when the pediatrician is equally hurried.

Indirect psychological consultation also takes the form of didactic lectures or case conferences. In my experience, didactic presentations are most effective and well received if they stem from a pragmatic need that is identified by pediatricians (e.g., how do we recognize a child with a learning disability and what do we do about it?) and if they include ample case material and practical suggestions for pediatric management (see Chapter 3). Case conferences that are focused on interesting diagnostic dilemmas or difficult but potentially soluble clinical management problems are also well received. Case presentations with a teaching moral, e.g., that illustrate success stories of positive management outcomes and model interdisciplinary collaboration, are also instructive. On the other hand, a sure-fire way to make a pediatrician's eyes glaze over, engender drowsiness, and reduce collective heart rates and enthusiasm for psychology is to discuss psychological theory or a body of research without clearly identifying the clinical relevance and "take-home" message for pediatric care. Many pediatricians, especially those in training, are not enchanted by presentations of complex, insoluble clinical problems because they engender feelings of helplessness (Duff, Rowe, & Anderson, 1972).

In my experience, indirect consultation is most effective if it involves continuing interactions between pediatricians and psychologists on management of clinical problems (see Chapters 3, 4, 14, and 15). Some pediatric psychologists have met the challenge of practical relevance by developing treatment instructions for parents and practitioners and summarizing research information, diagnostic issues, and treatment recommendations for various problems (Christophersen, 1982; Roberts, 1986).

Like any single model, the indirect model of consultation is not without its drawbacks. Some pediatricians may become impatient with the psychologist's teaching and/or supervisory methods because they want immediate results. Moreover, it may not always be possible to generate practical solutions to complex clinical problems that can be readily implemented by pediatricians without fostering illusions (Drotar, 1983). Some psychologists also become disenchanted with teaching pediatricians because they feel that they cannot provide in-depth, psychologically minded presentations.

The indirect or process-educative consultation model is also extremely time consuming for the pediatrician and psychologist and hence is readily replaced by more familiar direct service models. For example, as psychologists become busier in providing direct service to pediatric patients, which is an inevitable byproduct of successful consultation, they have less time to teach. Hence, very careful structuring of time is needed to ensure an adequate balance of direct service and indirect consultation methods.

Collaborative Team Model

A third generic model of consultation, the collaborative team model, is characterized by shared responsibility and joint decision making among psychologists, pediatricians, and other professionals (Roberts, 1986). Collaborative team models may be an integral part of some settings, e.g., programs for interdisciplinary care of children with developmental disabilities in university-affiliated centers. Effective collaborative team consultation cannot be forced or legislated but evolves among individuals who have worked together effectively over time and gradually negotiate their roles and working styles (Stabler, 1988). The essence of collaborative team consultation is a sharing of the expertise of different disciplines in clinical management, research, or teaching roles. Team members can benefit a great deal from such sharing and may eventually change their typical modes of functioning to operate in new ways (Drotar & Sturm, in press). For example, a pediatrician may learn to "think like a social worker" in obtaining family history and bringing in other family members to formulate a management plan. Psychologists learn to be savvy about differential medical diagnosis and to consider relevant medical factors in evaluating physical or psychological symptoms.

The challenge in this kind of consultation is for team members to learn from one another and extend their repertoire of professional skills while preserving their unique professional and personal contributions to the team. In my experience, organization and leadership of a team are critical to successful collaborative team consultation. Without suitable structures for agenda setting and problem solving, a team can easily become mired in dissension and indecision. On the other hand, autocratic leadership that squelches shared problem solving delivers deadly blows to collaborative teams.

Perhaps the major downside of the team model is the time that is needed. Moreover, it is difficult to fund interdisciplinary teams in the cost-conscious atmosphere of modern pediatric hospitals. Finally, collaborative team consultation makes taxing personal demands on sharing of responsibilities, communication, and flexibility of role functioning.

Systems Approach

The models of consultation discussed thus far emphasize interactions and relationships among the psychologist, pediatrician, and/or other professionals. However, a final model, the systems-oriented perspective, considers the impact of the broader context in which collaborative relations occur. Mullins *et al.* (1992) described the importance of planning interventions at several different levels and involve multiple professionals and family members and present a useful, detailed case illustration of this approach. In the present volume, the systems perspectives and team collaboration are emphasized in Chapters 4, 5, and 9. A systems perspective can be used to develop new and more optimal patterns and settings of care delivery and professional roles (Ack, 1974; Tefft & Simmeonsson, 1979).

Although pediatric psychologists have not written extensively about their involvement in creation of new settings or programs, Ack's (1974) description of his work in helping to design the environment of a new hospital is a classic example. In his new position as Director of Mental Health, Ack was asked by the Board of Trustees and physicians at Minneapolis Children's Medical Center to help design a hospital program where children's emotional needs would be given as much weight as their physical status. Ack and his colleagues convened a volunteer committee including community professionals and staff. A key element of the philosophy of this program, which one can only envy in the modern era of cost accountability, was the balancing of economic and patient care needs at every level. This led to a strong emphasis on parental participation in children's care, e.g., unlimited visiting privileges for parents and siblings, including accompanying children to anesthesia, parental rooming in, routine preoperative tours and preparation for children undergoing surgery, special rooms for privacy, and various design and architectural innovations designed to humanize the hospital environment. Moreover, psychologists were involved in interviewing and hiring all supervisory personnel to assess their capacity to work with children and in giving seminars in the psychology of leadership, regularly scheduled mental health care conferences, and seminars for other hospital staff on topics such as psychology of stress and psychological effects of hospitalization.

To my mind, one of the most impressive features of Ack's (1974) organizational restructuring was the assignment of 50% of the mental health professionals' time, including psychiatrists, social workers, and psychologists, to preventive services in the hospital. Recently M. Ack (personal communication, Feb. 18, 1994) noted that although many of the general environmental features, e.g., preparation of children for surgery, of his initial design are still intact, mental health services have become much more limited.

The systems approach to consultation has conceptual elegance and intuitive appeal and opens up opportunities for creating the type of change that can make traditional patient-centered consultation pale by comparison. For example, a systems perspective can facilitate the development of novel clinical services that address the relationship of hospital-based and community services. Not surprisingly, the major drawback of this approach is the difficulty of implementing this model. There are so many different systems-related problems at so many different levels that even the most conscientious and dedicated devotees of this approach can feel overwhelmed. The systems approach's strongest point is in many ways its weakest: it involves the efforts of multiple people in multiple settings.

Influences on Collaborative Outcomes

Pediatric psychologists' descriptions of models of consultation with physicians have outstripped their understanding of the factors that influence collaborative outcomes. Although it is difficult to define outcomes, such parameters as frequency of referrals or physicians' satisfaction with psychological services are examples (Olson, Holden, Friedman, Faust, Kenning, & Mason, 1988). One might also define a collaborative outcome as the degree to which it benefits the child or family, i.e., leads to improved clinical outcome (Charlop, Parrish, Fenton, & Cataldo, 1987). The frequency and/or quality of collaborative products that result from teaching (e.g., development of a new curriculum, rotation for residents) or research (e.g., collaborative grant proposal or publications) are other examples of products that can be used as a rough and ready index of the success of collaboration (see Chapter 10 for a review of empirical studies).

Pediatric psychologists have been hampered by limited models of the factors that influence the process and outcomes of collaboration. On the basis of observations of the culture of medical settings (Freidson, 1970; Mechanic, 1978), descriptions of collaboration (Stabler, 1988; Drotar, 1983), and models of influences on behavior in health settings (Becker, 1974), I have proposed several factors that might be expected to influence collaborators' initial decisions to work together as well as outcomes (Drotar, 1993), as shown in Table 2. These include the following: (1) participants' beliefs about the need for and expectations of collaborative outcomes; (2) participants' knowledge, skills, and prior experience in collaborative activities; and (3) setting-based barriers and supports.

Beliefs and Expectations Concerning Collaboration

I would hypothesize that a pediatrician's decision to request help from a psychologist or other professional colleague is influenced by the following beliefs and/or expectations: (1) belief that a particular clinical or research problem cannot be managed as effectively if it is done independently; (2) expectation that another professional can help to manage this problem; and (3) belief that this colleague's help is accessible. One would

Table 2. Influences on Collaborative Outcomes

Beliefs/Expectations	*Skills*	*Situational Incentives/Constraint*
Belief that collaboration is necesary, effective, or accessible	Problem identification	Accessibility
Beliefs about collaborative roles and authority	Making effective requests and use of information	Time pressures
	Communication and interpersonal skills	Multiple responsibilities
		Funding patterns
		Reimbursibility patterns
		Administrative organization

↓

Collaborative Outcomes

Frequency	*Efficacy/Quality*
Physician utilization of psychological services	Perceived benefits and satisfaction
Collaborative research and teaching	More efficient patient care
Mutual consultation	Economic benefits
	Publications

From *Journal of Pediatric Psychology, Vol. 18,* 1993, p. 164.

also expect that the decision to contact a colleague for help is facilitated by a belief that the potential benefits of this action, e.g., improved patient care, will outweigh the perceived costs of a collaborative action, e.g., time and effort involved in making the referral. For example, in order to ask for help with a clinical problem, the pediatrician must first identify a significant problem based on observation, history, etc. Physicians may identify problems but will not refer them if they believe that they can manage them independently. They will not initiate collaboration unless they believe that a problem's outcome can be enhanced by input, e.g., a clinical opinion, or action by another profession. Finally, the pediatrician must identify a specific professional (among many possibilities) who he or she believes can be helpful with a particular clinical problem and who is accessible (Bergman & Fritz, 1985). Even though a pediatrician believes that a particular professional is highly competent, that pediatrician will not request help if it does not appear to be readily obtainable.

A different set of beliefs and expectations may be necessary to maintain cooperative activities once they are initiated. Following initial contact with a colleague, collaborators may review their experience by asking themselves questions such as, "Was this person accessible and easy to work with?" "Was this an effective intervention?" "What did this family think of the intervention?" If participants judge their efforts as reasonably successful, they may decide to work together again. On the other hand, if their expectations are not met, subsequent requests or contacts may be limited or even abandoned.

The model that I am proposing suggests that both psychologists and physicians judge the success of a particular collaborative effort on the basis of *implicit* (but not necessarily realistic) expectations about how the other *should* perform in their respective collegial roles (Stabler & Murray, 1973). For example, in keeping with the traditional medical consultation model, physicians expect their psychologist colleagues to provide prompt and specific feedback based on their evaluation, effective treatment recommendations, and, in some cases, follow-up for their patients (Olson *et al.*, 1988) and may become dissatisfied when their expectations are violated (Meyer, Fink, & Carey, 1988) (see Chapter 10). Because such expectations are not necessarily realistic and are not verbalized, they may be sources of collaborative tension. For example, pediatricians' expectations concerning collaborative roles and authority and models of the etiology and treatment of clinical problems (Katon & Kleinman, 1981), which influence their expectations of how problems should be managed, are strongly rooted in profession-specific models of training and practice (Fox, 1957; Freidson, 1970).

Collaborative Skills and Knowledge

Interprofessional collaboration requires considerable skills and knowledge, many of which are not explicitly taught in training programs. For example, in order for a pediatrician to utilize his or her professional counterpart most effectively, he or she must not only identify problems that are suitable for psychological management but make requests that are clear, feasible, and fit with a colleague's skills. The ability to utilize information from one's collaborators effectively is another important attribute. Skilled psychological consultants learn to translate information from their assessment into specific recommendations that can be effectively utilized by their pediatric colleagues (Stabler, 1988).

One of the more interesting but least understood questions concerns the way in which professionals' knowledge, skills, and beliefs about collaboration are modified by collaborative experiences in training and on the job (Drotar, 1993). One possibility is that a positive collaborative experience helps to transform a more general stereotypic view of other professionals (e.g., psychologists are useful for assessment but not therapy) to a more differentiated one (e.g., psychologist X has been helpful to me in managing cases of encopresis). On the other hand, unsuccessful experiences that fall short of expectations might stimulate more negative generalizations; e.g., psychologists are just not practical; pediatricians are concrete, especially for inexperienced collaborators. The skills that are necessary to establish and maintain successful collaborative relationships are also not well understood, but attributes such as respect for colleagues, a strong interest in mutual learning, and interpersonal skills may be critical (Davidson, 1988; Stabler, 1988; also see Epilogue)

Situational Incentives and Constraints

Situational incentives and constraints also have powerful effects on the quality of collaboration. Many pediatricians operate under a highly compressed time and action span in which the costs and benefits of all clinical actions, including collaboration, must be carefully measured. The pressures of practice reward an economy-of-effort orientation that emphasizes rapid appraisal and disposition of problems and limits the time for clinical or research collaborations. Such constraints heighten a pediatrician's need for accessible psychological consultants, a point that has been clearly recognized by many pediatric psychologists (Roberts, 1986; Schroeder & Mann, 1991; Stabler, 1988).

Psychologists also do not operate in a vacuum. Their accessibility to their pediatric colleagues may be severely limited by their other responsibilities. For this reason, in many settings, the quality of administrative organization and deployment of psychologists may be a key determinant of the quality of interprofessional collaboration over the long haul. Consequently, there is a compelling need to identify organizations and settings that promote effective interprofessional cooperation (see Chapter 8).

Importance of Professional Socialization

The models of consultation that have been described in this chapter underscore the need to consider the powerful role of professional socialization. Psychologists and physicians have each been highly socialized into their respective professional roles and models of problems and use very different languages in teaching, practice, and research. Psychologists and physicians tend to underestimate how much their communications reflect their profession-specific language and how much they can be misunderstood by those who are unfamiliar with their professions (Fox, 1957; Friedson, 1970; Stabler, 1988). Much of consultation can be seen as a way of bridging the many gaps in language, communication, and differing models that are heavily overlearned in the course of professional training. Successful psychological consultants have learned to make effective translations of their training and technical expertise that are utilizable by their physician colleagues in a range of settings. The information presented in many of the chapters in this book illustrates various ways of enhancing such translations.

IMPLICATIONS: ENHANCING COLLABORATIVE SUCCESS

The present model suggests that collaborative success will increase as a function of individual colleagues' skills, their beliefs in the efficacy of collaborative work, and the ratio of positive incentives to constraints on collaboration present in a particular setting. One strength of the present framework is that it suggests potential targets for interventions to enhance the frequency and/or quality of collaborative activities. Most but not all situational constraints are fixed conditions that are amenable to change only under exceptional circumstances, e.g., increased funding. On the other hand, professionals' beliefs, expectations, and skills related to collaboration could be enhanced by training that includes successful collaborative experiences with colleagues. For example, observation of mentors who engage in successful and personally satisfying interdisciplinary collaboration should help to modify unrealistic expectations of other professionals, especially if this is accompanied by supervised practice in interdisciplinary communication and consultation (see Chapter 11). Another option is for psychologists to develop services that minimize the barriers to collaboration. The collaborative practices described in Chapters 12 and 13 are good examples of this.

Another use of this framework is to help collaborators identify factors that might be interfering with their work and to consider possible interventions to enhance these efforts. For example, in some settings it may be possible to limit time constraints by allocating more time to a valued collaboration or developing a conjoint proposal for research funding or clinical services. Although it is very difficult to change fixed situational constraints, colleagues who can clearly identify specific obstacles to their work and communicate with one another about their impact should have less frustrating and/or blame-producing encounters.

Finally, this framework suggests several directions for research to extend the meager base of empirical work and develop this preliminary model. For example, naturalistic, observational research strategies that have been used by sociologists and anthropologists to study medical culture (Fox, 1957) provide useful descriptions of physicians' and psychologists' personal models of beliefs, expectations, and decision making concerning interdisciplinary collaboration. It would also be very helpful to describe the characteristics of settings where collaboration has evolved into comprehensive, programmatic efforts as compared with settings where this type of collaboration either has not developed or has been abandoned (see Chapter 8). Psychologists also need to devote more energies to describing and documenting the efficacy of collaboration (see Chapter 10).

The strongest inferences will be made from tests of specific interventions that are designed to enhance the frequency and/or quality of collaborative management of clinical problems (Drotar, 1993). Such interventions might be most effective if they focus on improving specific skills, e.g., problem identification, communication with other professionals, that are necessary for collaborative clinical management of problems that are frequently encountered in practice. Research that documents the practical benefits of collaboration to hospital administrators and pediatric colleagues is also necessary.

3

Consultation and Collaboration in Primary Care Settings

By virtue of their role in well-child care and child and health supervision, pediatricians and nurse practitioners in primary care settings are in an excellent position to identify and institute interventions that prevent or alleviate problems that threaten children's physical health and emotional well-being. Primary care refers to outpatient or ambulatory care that is provided to children who are not hospitalized. Pediatric psychologists' training and interests make for natural partnerships with pediatricians concerning the problems that present in primary care (Christophersen & Abernathy, 1982; Routh, Schroeder, & Koocher, 1983).

However, the potential for such collaboration has yet to be realized because of several factors. Despite improved coverage of behavioral and developmental problems in pediatric training (Davidson, 1988), pediatricians may not be well equipped to recognize and manage an increasingly complex array of problems. Even a short list of problems is daunting for the most psychologically minded of pediatricians, let alone for those less well endowed (AAP Committee on Psychosocial Aspects of Child and Family Health, 1993). Pediatricians are expected to recognize and manage developmental and behavioral problems, e.g., depression or learning and attention-deficit disorder, as well as a host of environmental threats: family violence, child abuse and neglect, and parenting and family relationship problems. In the course of a typical work day, pediatricians may conduct physical exams and take histories to assess acute medical problems, make decisions concerning treatment of fever, and decide whether to hospitalize a child who has possible meningitis. Moreover, they carry out preventive services including a wide range of screening, parent counseling, and immunization services (Report of U.S. Preventive Services Task Force, 1989).

Pediatric interventions may include supportive counseling for a child and family who are undergoing divorce, medication and behavioral management with a child with attention deficit with hyperactivity, or referral of a child to county welfare protective services for child abuse. Does this short list of activities sound overwhelming to you? It does to me.

Pediatricians' abilities to carry out such diverse practice agendas are affected by many constraints. Although the list of behavioral, psychological, and family problems that are under the pediatrician's purview has steadily grown, the basic demands of practice, e.g., health monitoring and supervision, preventive care, management of acute medical problems, and preventive guidance for parents, have not diminished. Along with their colleagues in medicine and psychology, pediatricians face the problems of shrinking reimbursement for ambulatory care services. This has forced pediatricians into a high-volume practice where the average length of an office visit is 10–15 minutes (Bergman, Dassel, & Wedgewood, 1966). How much early identification, developmental anticipatory guidance, and emotional support can be packed into a 10- to 15-minute office visit without giving short shrift to the assessment of child's health status?

Collaborative involvement of pediatric psychologists might help to address these problems (Schroeder & Mann, 1991). However, many pediatricians do not have access to psychologists who are trained to provide services that are compatible with primary care settings. Other important but unanswered questions concerning collaborative management in primary care include the following: which problems should pediatricians manage? Which are effectively managed by other professions? What are the most optimal ways for psychologists and pediatricians in ambulatory care to work together?

This chapter describes a broad range of issues related to consultation and collaboration between psychologists and pediatricians in primary care settings. These include service delivery, teaching pediatricians in primary care settings, guidelines and issues in consultation in outpatient settings, models of consultation in community practice settings, and collaborative research in primary care. In this chapter, particular emphasis is placed on consultation in primary care settings in academic medical settings because I am most familiar with such settings. Collaborative pediatric practice in community settings is also considered in Chapters 12 and 13.

REFERRAL PROBLEMS AND SERVICES IN PRIMARY CARE SETTINGS

The referral problems and psychological services that are provided in primary care differ substantially from those that are encountered in inpatient settings (see Chapter 4). Roberts (1986) compared referral patterns reported in three different ambulatory care settings, a pediatric clinic serving a large children's hospital (Walker, 1979), a private pediatric practice (Kanoy & Schroeder, 1985), and a pediatric psychology practicum in a clinical training program (Ottinger & Roberts, 1980). As sorted into problem categories developed by Mesibov, Schroeder, and Wesson (1977), consistent patterns of referral problems were encountered across the three settings. The most frequently noted referral problems included (1) negative behaviors, e.g., oppositional, tantrums, demanding behavior; (2) toileting problems, e.g., enuresis and encopresis; (3) developmental delays; (4) school problems; and (5) personality problems, e.g., lack of self control and irresponsibility. Infrequently referred problems include understanding and adjusting to death, guidance of gifted and talented children, gender identity problems, and specific fears (e.g., dogs). However, differences in referral patterns across settings were also noted. For example, physical complaints, e.g., headaches, stomachache, were among the problems that were referred most frequently to the psychology practicum facility (Ottinger & Roberts, 1980) and a pediatric clinic in a children's hospital (Walker, 1979) but were rarely referred in the pediatric private practice (Kanoy & Schroeder, 1985).

Comparable referral patterns have been noted in more recent descriptions. For example, Charlop, Parrish, Fenton, and Cataldo (1987) described referral problems of 100 patients who received behavioral treatment during a 1-year period at a university-based pediatric psychology service. Parents ranked behavioral noncompliance (16.2%), tantrums (12.8%), and aggression (8.1%) as the top three behaviors of greatest concern. Other behaviors that were ranked highly by parents included self-injurious behavior, feeding problems, and elimination disorders.

Similarly, among Finney, Riley, and Cataldo's (1991) series of 93 children referred for psychological treatment in a university-based health maintenance organization (HMO), the largest group (56%) were referred for behavioral problems, e.g., aggression, tantrums, noncompliance, sleep, and mealtime problems. Children with toileting problems, e.g., enuresis and encopresis (16%), and psychosomatic problems (20%), e.g., recurrent abdominal pain, headaches, tics, or obesity, were also referred frequently.

CONSULTATION IN PRIMARY CARE ACADEMIC MEDICAL SETTINGS

Structuring Service Delivery

Given the nature and volume of referral problems described above, service provision is an important component of a pediatric psychology consultation service in primary care. However, psychologists in academic ambulatory care settings also provide a broad range of teaching and research functions and may also consult to other services as well. Consequently, they need to prioritize their services carefully so that they do not get swallowed up by providing ongoing treatment for large numbers of children. In some settings, for example, it may be possible to focus on developing services for a subgroup of children with compelling clinical and/or teaching needs, e.g., children with attention deficit with hyperactivity disorder (ADHD).

Given the extraordinary needs for psychological services in primary care settings, psychological consultants need to carefully clarify and negotiate the type and nature of services, e.g., assessment versus intervention, that will be provided, how much time will be given to service, and how their other activities will be deployed. The high volume of referrals underscores the need for consultants in primary care settings to develop close links with community agencies and to become familiar with available services for children with a range of psychological problems. Psychologists in primary care settings need to consider carefully how they allocate time to clinical service versus other activities, in order to ensure that they maximize their opportunities for teaching.

Teaching Pediatricians in Primary Care Settings

Pediatric residents in primary care settings see children with highly prevalent developmental, learning, and behavioral problems that provide important teaching opportunities about early identification and clinical management. In some of these settings, psychologists have assumed a high level of initiative and leadership roles in the development of teaching and training in the behavioral and developmental aspects of pediatric practice (Stancin, Constantinou, & Walker, 1989). To maximize the efficiency of such teaching, psychologists need to be very available to residents and hence to spend a considerable amount of time in the clinic setting.

A wide range of teaching methods are utilized in primary care academic medical settings (see Chapters 14 and 15). For example, to enhance both teaching and clinical service, some psychologists find it useful to meet directly with the child and/or parent to obtain some information history immediately following a consultation request from a resident (Salk, 1970). In such instances, a case disposition, e.g., psychological assessment, can be quickly arranged and discussed with the pediatrician. This kind of clinical triage can also enhance parental compliance with follow-up because family members appreciate the opportunity to associate a face with a referral and discuss their concerns about their child and expectations for the assessment. The obvious downside of this "on the spot" model is that the consultant may not be able to devote blocks of dedicated time without compromising his or her other responsibilities.

Irrespective of the specific teaching model that is employed, some pediatric residents have difficulty accepting teaching, supervision, and/or consultation from psychologists (see Chapters 14 and 15) unless it is strongly supported and modeled by pediatric faculty. One model of teaching that has some utility is on-the-spot precepting or case supervision. The essence of this approach is the opportunity for the resident to discuss a child whom he or she has just seen with multiple faculty members. Terry Stancin (personal communication, Nov. 12, 1993) has effectively employed such a model in a university-based primary care setting at Metrohealth Medical Center in Cleveland. Stancin's primary role involves teaching pediatricians interviewing and prevention, assessment, and intervention in primary care. In this role, she works closely with a nurse practitioner who assists pediatricians with basic well-child care issues and coordinates didactic conferences and faculty pediatricians. To ensure optimal responsiveness to pediatric residents, Stancin does not typically provide a great deal of direct service to patients but functions as liaison to other resources in the hospital and community.

In this setting, residents are divided among four afternoon continuity care clinics. Each resident is expected to see four to eight patients per afternoon for well-child or follow-up visits. This is a culturally and ethnically diverse patient population and includes a large number of infants and young children from indigent or working poor families. The continuity care clinic uses a team precepting approach in which teaching and supervision responsibilities are shared by general pediatricians, a pediatric psychologist, and a nurse practitioner. Thus, the psychologist's teaching role is an integral part of the model of pediatric training and is supported by pediatric faculty. The way that this model works is shown in the following example.

Dr. A, a second year resident, has just seen a 3-year-old child for a well-child care visit and returned to the clinic conference room for precepting. The resident noted that the child has several potential problems. She is well below the 10th percentile in weight and height and the 10th percentile in head circumference. The child's language was also delayed, based on assessment using the Denver Developmental Screening Test. Medical history was significant for a previously diagnosed heart murmur and a hospitalization in another state at 9 months of age for failure to thrive (FTT). As the child's history was presented to the pediatric faculty preceptor, the psychologist was called to listen as well. The pediatrician discussed additional information that the resident should obtain, including a diet history, previous measurements, laboratory tests, etc. The psychologist advised the resident to obtain additional developmental, behavioral, and social information from the child's mother. Ten minutes later, the resident returned to report that the family has been sent to the lab for blood work and that an additional interview with the mother indicated that the child has significant behavioral problems: she refuses to eat meals but instead "grazes" on snacks and fruit juice. Moreover, she is "unable" to fall asleep in her bed until 2:00–3:00 a.m., and her mother lies in bed with her until then. With input from all preceptors, an assessment and management plan were then outlined to address the following problem list that was generated: (1) FTT, (2) developmental delay, (3) sleep problems. The resident then followed up on each of these problems under supervision.

GUIDELINES FOR CLINICAL CONSULTATION IN PRIMARY CARE SETTINGS

The practice of clinical psychological consultation in primary care settings is similar to inpatient work (see Chapter 4) but raises some special issues that need to be considered.

Clarifying the Referral Request

Physicians in ambulatory care settings generally make referrals by a letter, which provides a helpful written record, or by phone. Irrespective of the specific methods of initial contact, it is important to clarify the nature of the referral question by phone or face-to-face contact. Given the time constraints on pediatricians, detailed, time-consuming questions about the child's medical or family history are not as productive as finding out precisely what the referring physician wants to find out about the child's psychological status. Similar to inpatient consultation requests, ambulatory care referral questions range from vague requests such as "the child needs psychometric testing" or "I'd like to know what you think about this child" (the projective request) to more specific and difficult questions such as, "This child is on a course of medication for his asthma. I'd like to know if this is affecting his learning and behavior".

Structuring Referral Procedures

Referral procedures vary as a function of the specific primary care setting (see Hurley and Cunningham, Chapters 12 and 13). In most instances, the parents of the child who is referred for psychological consultation will make the initial contact by phone. However, in some settings, physicians will "send" the parents directly to the office to make the appointment. Moreover, some residents, in particular, may want the psychologist to make the initial contact with the family because they feel that this will ensure compliance with the consultation.

In teaching hospitals where very large numbers of pediatric faculty and residents refer patients, establishing specific procedures for making referrals will often reduce the disruption and confusion caused by multiple referral sources. For this reason, a *brief* referral form containing information concerning the child's presenting problem, the physician's referral questions, and relevant medical or family background information may be useful. To make the procedure even more pediatrician-friendly, information can be recorded based on a phone or face-to-face contact. Irrespective of how referral information is obtained, a record should be maintained so that the status of referrals can be tracked, e.g., if the family misses appointments. There is a fine and difficult line between imposing sufficient structure on the referral process to maximize efficiency of follow-up and developing cumbersome, bureaucratic procedures that increase frustration among pediatric colleagues and reduce their zeal to refer.

Repeated lectures and discussions are generally needed to clarify how best to make referrals to pediatric psychology and to inform house staff and faculty about the availability of services. Such teaching conferences also serve the purpose of increasing pediatric colleagues' awareness of psychological services in their setting, enhancing their knowledge about screening and early recognition of psychological problems, and helping them to decide which problems should be referred.

Discussing the Referral with Family Members

As in inpatient settings, one encounters varying levels of parental acceptance and understanding of psychological referrals in primary care settings. Some parents have only minimal information and understanding of the referral and may note only that their child's doctor wanted them to come in to the psychologist. Others may misunderstand the purpose of the referral. It is not uncommon for parents to express questions and concerns about their child's behavior or development that are discrepant from pediatricians' views, e.g., parents who do not feel the child's problems are significant or describe problems that are very different from their pediatrician's concerns. Consequently, as part of every consultation, it is very useful to review the parents' understanding of their child's problems and their understanding of the purpose of the psychological assessment and to discuss with them and their children the specific procedures that will be done and how their pediatrician will be involved in management.

Giving Feedback to Pediatricians

Similar to their colleagues everywhere, pediatricians in ambulatory care settings place a high value on the clarity and speed of the psychologist's communications to them concerning their patients. Follow-up notes to pediatricians in primary care should clearly and briefly communicate what was done in the psychological evaluation, findings and impressions, recommendations, and information about the psychologist's role in follow-up. The extended "full battery" test report that psychologists learn to write in training is simply not appropriate for most pediatricians, who will not only not have time to read it but may be frustrated by the plethora of information that it may contain. In writing such notes, I have found a conversational tone and "just the facts" approach to be helpful. However, one might include more detail for pediatric house staff to enhance the teaching value of the consultation. The following is an example of such a note that was sent to a pediatrician concerning a child who was referred for behavioral problems:

> Dear Dr. (or first name if a familiar colleague):
>
> This is a note to give you feedback concerning my recent evaluation of Don T, age 6. As you know, Mrs. T has been concerned about many areas of her son's behavior. One of her main concerns has been his lying, which occurs not only with her but with his peers. According to her, Don has trouble accepting responsibility for something he has done and will tell tall tales in order to get attention from others. Not surprisingly, this behavior has had the opposite effect, as he has had trouble making friends. Finally, Don reportedly has difficulty accepting even basic responsibilities for doing things (e.g., picking up his clothes) independently. These problems have caused considerable conflict between Don and his mother and in the family in general. Mrs. T reports that she has difficulty communicating with Don, who is by far the youngest of her three children and the only boy. She is very frustrated that he doesn't listen to her and wonders whether he might have an attention deficit disorder.
>
> For this evaluation, I interviewed Don and his parents and conducted psychological testing. My interviews with Don indicated that he is a bright but somewhat disorganized boy who was defensive about his problems. He preferred to cover over what appear to be considerable insecurities by telling exciting stories in which he was always the hero. In conversation, he tends to be very controlling. I would think that this behavior might interfere with his peer relationships. In general, I found him to be socially and emotionally immature. However, based on testing, observation, and information from his parents and teacher, I did not see any signs of a clinically significant attention deficit disorder.
>
> Although my evaluation did not indicate a serious emotional disturbance, Don's behavior is certainly troubling to his parents and interferes with his relationship with them. For this reason, the family would benefit from a brief intervention of parent guidance involving behavior management. In a follow-up session, Mrs. T was quite

accepting of this plan. She is anxious to do whatever she can to prevent Don from developing more psychological problems and to understand him better. The plan will also involve Mr. T in parent guidance as his schedule permits. Thank you for the referral. I will keep you informed concerning his progress.

In my experience, pediatricians value psychologists who provide continuity of care and prompt, relevant help to their patients and their families. In addition to written notes, some pediatricians may appreciate a phone call to touch base. Experienced consultants will also provide more detailed case discussion to house staff as part of their education. Individual pediatricians have varying styles about how they prefer to receive feedback. I remember going out of my way to give detailed information to a faculty surgeon who had made several referrals of outpatients. His reply to my prompt, "relevant" feedback was something like: "What's the matter, don't you know I trust you?"

However, most pediatricians are generally very interested in obtaining follow-up information concerning the child's progress in psychological intervention and additional information about the child's problem and/or suggestions concerning management that become apparent after further diagnostic or therapeutic work. When the consultant makes recommendations, e.g., for medical management, that involve the pediatrician, additional dialogue will often be necessary.

Other Consultation Methods

Experienced consultants may utilize a range of methods to enhance teaching and clinical care in primary care settings. For example, developing specific behavior modification plans that can be carried out in collaboration with the physician is an important function. (Christophersen & Abernathy, 1982). In some situations, psychologist and pediatricians can work as cointerviewers and/or cotherapists (see Chapters 14 and 15). This type of clinical collaboration can be very effective but requires an excellent working alliance, high levels of communication, and low levels of defensiveness on both sides.

Psychologists who work with pediatricians in ambulatory care settings generally use a flexible range of interventions such as brief therapy, crisis intervention, intermittent contacts on an "as-needed" basis, or less frequent follow-up on a monthly or biweekly schedule of visits (Drotar *et al.*, 1982). In my experience, long-term, intermittent psychological follow-up can be an especially useful model in working with children with chronic physical problems or developmental problems who may need supportive help at times of crises or anticipatory guidance to manage an upcoming change, e.g., transition to school, or adolescent issues. In this model of follow-up, the psychologist operates in many ways more like a pediatrician or family practitioner (Vane & DeMaria, 1988).

Psychological Consultation in Community Pediatric Practice: Schroeder and Her Colleagues' Collaborative Practice Model

Psychological consultation in ambulatory community settings raises very special clinical and collaborative issues. Carolyn Schroeder and her colleagues' work in a private practice community setting is widely regarded as a model of psychological consultation and collaboration and bears some discussion. As it has continued for more than 20 years, this work is an outstanding example of programmatic collaboration that integrates clinical care, teaching, and research (Kanoy & Schroeder, 1985; Schroeder, 1979; Schroeder, Goolsby, & Stangler, 1975; Schroeder & Mann, 1991).

Schroeder (1979) noted that her collaboration with the only private pediatric office in Chapel Hill, North Carolina, that served 11,000 to 12,000 children began with and still has the primary goal of offering parents timely information, education, and intervention concerning their child's development. Concerned that young parents in our society are quite distant from relatives and friends and often do not know what to expect from their children, Schroeder and her colleagues, Elaine Goolsby and Sharon Stangler (1975), planned their initial program to address parents' educational needs concerning child development. From the outset, this was a collaborative effort with pediatricians in the practice.

To document the need for this service, Schroeder *et al.* (1975) conducted a telephone survey of parents who used the practice to ask them what concerns or problems they were having with their children and how they would like their concerns answered. Based on this information, services that were developed included the following: a call-in hour twice a week for 2 hours, a come-in service (4 hours a week), and parents' groups that were held three evenings a month. The come-in service allowed parents to have more of an in-depth discussion of a problem and also included students as participants. Although most appointments were arranged ahead of time through the practice, parents could also walk in to discuss a problem. Initial call-ins and come-ins averaged between 250 and 300 per year (Schroeder, 1979). Evening (1½-hour) parents' groups held in the pediatric office waiting room focused on either a particular age group (e.g., 1 week to 6 months, adolescence) or on topics (e.g., sibling rivalry, divorce) that cut across various ages.

One of several exemplary features of this practice was the fact that assessment of parental concerns, services, efficacy, and feasibility of intervention models was built into the practice from the outset. This research is described in more detail in Chapter 10. A record was kept of every patient contact, the age of the referred child and siblings, the stated problems, and the response. Daily logs of each contact with parents were also recorded. Parents were also asked at the end of each visit if they would participate in a follow-up call several months later. Very few refused this offer.

It should be noted that this data collection strategy provides a way for psychological consultants in ambulatory care settings to track the nature of presenting problems that are seen, changes in services that are offered over time, and consumer satisfaction. Such data are also very helpful in describing psychological services to pediatric colleagues and planning changes to enhance parental satisfaction. Such assessment of the nature and quality of clinical care is likely to become increasingly important when managed care takes hold (see Chapter 16).

Initially, services were offered free of charge because of training funds. Payments were required as the service evolved, and the practice has proven to be economically viable. Readers who are interested in the fiscal and management issues in setting up an independent practice of pediatric psychology should consult Schroeder and Mann (1991) and Chapter 12.

The current practice brochure (C. Schroeder, personal communication, Nov. 14, 1993) reflects the growth of the service and lists eight physicians in pediatric and adolescent medicine, four Ph.D.-level clinical psychologists, a Ph.D.-level educational psychologist, a master's-level child development specialist, a master's-level social worker, and a child psychiatrist. Psychological services that are currently offered include traditional individual diagnostic and treatment services along with agency consultation, therapeutic groups for children, and parents with similar concerns, e.g., coping with divorce, enhancing social skills, child behavioral management classes, a parent reference library, and an ADHD clinic that provides a full range of services including consultation to teachers. The free call-in hour for parents has been retained.

Schroeder and her colleagues' work is noteworthy not only for innovations in service delivery in ambulatory care but for the creative integration of training and research activities (Schroeder *et al.*, 1974). From the beginning of the practice, students from psychology, nursing, social work, psychiatry, pediatrics, and family medicine were trained in the call-in and come-in service. Schroeder's faculty status and collaboration with programs at the University of North Carolina School of Medicine undoubtedly facilitated the development of interdisciplinary teaching programs, including some that addressed the need for pediatricians to develop skills to manage childhood behavioral and developmental problems. In 1984, this teaching program was recognized by the American Academy of Ambulatory Pediatrics' Teaching Excellence Award. Medical students and residents each spend one day a week for a month in the practice learning about the developmental and behavioral concerns of parents, appropriate interviewing and interventions, the psychologist's contribution to clinical management, and when and how to refer (Schroeder & Mann, 1991). Clinical psychology graduate students have continued to participate in the call-in hour and provide treatment one afternoon a week. More recently, a 2-year postdoctoral fellow was sponsored by the practice and the University of North Carolina.

Finally, Schroeder and her colleagues have demonstrated the potential of a collaborative practice to provide consultation for community services and advocacy for children and their families. For example, the practice has become the coordinator for all the community agencies involved with children who were physically or sexually abused. Regular meetings focused on education and case management have been held with representatives from the pediatric office, police department, schools, and department of social services together with mental health professionals from the community. This work led to a contract to provide group treatment for children who have been sexually abused. The practice has also provided consultation to the local school system to include sex education and sex abuse prevention at all grade levels, training for the North Carolina guardian *ad litem* program, district court judges, district attorneys, department of social services, the rape crisis center, and day care centers. Hence, this practice has been a catalyst for services that positively affect the lives of children and families in the community.

COLLABORATIVE RESEARCH IN PRIMARY CARE SETTINGS

The founders of pediatric psychology clearly recognized the importance of advancing the scientific knowledge base concerning the management and prevention of the highly prevalent behavioral and developmental problems seen in pediatric practice (Kagan, 1965; Wright, 1967). Primary care settings are the central site for such collaborative research. However, as psychologists who work in these sites can attest, it is very difficult to conduct research at these sites given the heavy practice demands (see Chapter 12 and 13). Nevertheless, psychologists have made consistent and significant contributions to research in these settings, which will be briefly described here. Research in primary care settings that pertains more directly to evaluation of consultation and collaboration will be reviewed in Chapter 10.

Schroeder and her colleagues' clinical research has been integrated into service activities throughout the history of their practice (Kanoy & Schroeder, 1985; Schroeder, Gordon, Kanoy, & Routh, 1983). However, research in the practice has evolved from a primary emphasis on service evaluation to include assessment of parent training for nonconcompliance, knowledge of sexuality in normal and sexually abused children (Gordon, Schroeder, & Abrams, 1990 a,b), and children's memory of physical examination (Baker-Ward, Gordon, Omstein, Larus, & Clubb, 1993).

Christophersen and his colleagues at the University of Kansas and elsewhere have developed exemplary models for the application of behavioral interventions to pediatric care in many areas: childbirth education classes, course on child development, behavioral management, discipline, accident prevention, etc. (Christophersen, 1982, 1983, 1991, 1992, 1993; Christophersen & Abernathy, 1982; Rapoff & Christophersen, 1982). Moreover, this work has developed guidelines for pediatricians to utilize in providing guidance to parents concerning common problems such as dressing, mealtime, bedtime, toileting, and behavioral problems.

Another important body of work by Christophersen and his colleagues has concerned prevention, especially accident prevention. This work is exemplary in its clinical application and high level of initiative and ingenuity. For example, Christophersen and Gyulay (1981) developed and tested the effectiveness of detailed written notes that instructed parents how to introduce car seats, to utilize them, and the importance of verbally attending to children in the car. According to a multiple-baseline across-subjects design and an ecologically valid measurement (direct observation during automobile rides), a significant reduction in the frequency of children's inappropriate behaviors in cars was demonstrated. Moreover, these results were maintained on 12-month follow-up. Christophersen, Sosland-Edelman, and LeClaire (1985) have also evaluated the efficacy of infant car seat loaner programs.

Development of programs that enhance the efficacy of pediatricians' interventions by using behavioral methods are an important next frontier of collaborative research. The results of pediatric interventions such as well-child care and anticipatory guidance, designed to enhance children's health, behavior, and development, have been reviewed elsewhere (Christophersen, 1982; Christophersen & Abernathy, 1982; Schroeder *et al.*, 1983). One such study involved a collaboration between a pediatrician (Casey) and a pediatric psychologist (Whitt) to test the efficacy of pediatric guidance in well-child care (Whitt & Casey 1982). Thirty mothers and healthy first-born infants seen in five well-child visits from 2 to 21 weeks of age were randomly assigned to a control group, who received customary care, or to an intervention group, who, in addition, received guidance that was based on the infant's developmental status. Intervention-group mothers were rated more highly on sensitivity, cooperation, appropriateness of interaction, and appropriateness of play. In addition, infants whose mothers received the intervention had more advanced vocal imitation.

More recently, pediatric psychologists have assessed the effectiveness of behavioral strategies in improving health care compliance and parent–provider interaction. For example, using a randomized design, Finney, Friman, Rapoff, and Christophersen (1986) found that compliance enhancement strategies (self-monitoring, calendar, and telephone reminders) improved compliance with antibiotic regimen for otitis media. Reminders and parking passes have also been shown to enhance compliance with appointments for routine pediatric care (Friman, Finney, Rapoff, & Christophersen, 1985). Finally, strategies of prompting parents to initiate discussions of their concerns increased the frequency of parents' interactions and discussion of behavioral and health topics with pediatricians and nurse providers during young children's health supervision visits (Finney, Brophy, Friman, Golden, Richman, & Ross, 1990). This research clearly illustrates how psychological science can be used to enhance the quality and efficiency of pediatric care.

4

Consultation and Collaboration in Pediatric Inpatient Settings

Pediatric psychologists are often asked to consult with pediatricians concerning the problems of hospitalized children and adolescents. This type of consultation raises special issues that will be considered in this chapter. Interested readers should also consult Christophersen and Long (1987) or Huszti and Walker (1991) for useful descriptions.

REFERRAL PROBLEMS/SERVICES IN INPATIENT SETTINGS

Although specific referrals of hospitalized children vary with the setting, available data suggest some common features. My survey of 528 hospitalized children and adolescents who were referred to a new pediatric psychology service over a 3-year period at Rainbow Babies and Children's Hospital in Cleveland identified several common referral problems (Drotar, 1977a). These included assessment of cognitive development (n = 243) for children with presumed developmental delay, psychological adaptation to chronic disease and handicap (n = 104), the role of psychological factors in physical symptoms (n = 92), evaluation of behavioral problems (n = 48), and management of psychological crises (n = 41). A wide range of assessment and intervention services were utilized in the management of these referrals. The most challenging and time-consuming referrals involved the management of adolescent suicide attempts, depression, especially among children and adolescents with chronic physical illness, and adjustment to physical trauma and illness, including terminal illness (Drotar, 1977a).

More recently, Olson *et al.* (1989) described referral patterns among a larger sample (n = 740) of hospitalized children to a more established pediatric psychology service at Oklahoma Health Sciences Center over a 4½-year period. The pattern of referral problems was somewhat different in this setting. For example, the largest number (n = 145) related to depression and suicide attempts. Relatively large numbers of children were also seen for adjustment to chronic illness (n = 92), behavioral problems (n = 69), psychosomatic problems (n = 61), and pain control (n = 57). Both surveys noted that relatively large numbers of referred children also had chronic physical problems. Differences in the referral problems in the two settings may have reflected differences in availability of other mental health services, e.g., child psychiatry, or the history of services (Huszti & Walker, 1991).

Each of the above surveys was conducted in large acute care hospitals in academic medical settings. Referral patterns are somewhat different in pediatric rehabilitation hospitals, another important resource for hospitalized children. For example, a survey of 127 consecutive referrals to a newly formed pediatric rehabilitation hospital (Singer & Drotar, 1989) identified large numbers of children with organic and nonorganic failure to thrive (FTT) (n = 46), neurological disorder (n = 26), developmental delay (n = 19), and psychophysiological disorders (n = 11). Many of these problems required specialized assessment for sensory and neuropsychological problems. Moreover, special consultation issues related to the active nature of staff's interventions and the chronicity of child and family problems.

Intervention and Follow-Up

Although many hospitalized children are referred to pediatric psychologists for assessment, many of these children also have problems that require more extended psychological intervention. In fact, pediatricians, nurses, and other staff expect that such follow-up will be provided. Olson *et al.* (1988) noted that over one-third of hospitalized children (37%) who were referred for psychological consultation on their service were seen once, 35% were seen two to four times, and 13% were seen extensively for more than 10 contacts as inpatients. This latter group required management of such compelling problems as terminal illness, burns, decannulation of tracheostomy, and eating disorders. We also identified a small subset of hospitalized children and adolescents with severe physical and/or psychological crises who required extensive psychological intervention (Drotar, 1977a).

Moreover, pediatric psychologists' work with hospitalized children does not necessarily end when the child is discharged. Olson *et al.* (1988) reported that 32% of hospitalized children seen for psychological consultation were subsequently followed as outpatients. Most of these patients were initially referred for depression or previous suicide attempts, adjustment to acute and chronic illness, and psychosomatic problems. Nearly a third were also referred to outside agencies for treatment (Olson *et al.*, 1988). The needs of hospitalized children for additional follow-up place considerable demands on pediatric psychologists to carve out time to provide some of these services and to become familiar with available community services.

Guidelines for Clinical Consultation with Hospitalized Children

Clarifying Referral Requests

Given the extraordinary time constraints of inpatient work, psychological consultants to such settings need to consider carefully how referrals to their service are screened and managed. For this reason, careful records of when the referral came in, when the referring person was contacted, and when the child was seen and by whom are essential. In some settings, referrals are made to the psychology service and then assigned to a specific consultant on the basis of availability or rotating assignments. In other settings, consultants not only are assigned to a specific division but are highly visible and have close, professional relationships with division staff (Geist, 1977). Such specialization has clear advantages for assessment and treatment planning but is very time consuming. Many psychology departments in pediatric hospitals simply do not have sufficient staff to provide such comprehensive coverage to inpatient services. Hence, the initial referral contact will often be made by phone, either to a particular consultant or to a central office. In some instances, medical staff will also fill out a consultation request form. I will usually encourage the staff to fill out the request form because this formalizes the procedure and encourages clarification of the referral.

In some instances, the problem for which the child was admitted to the hospital, e.g., FTT or a suicide attempt, will trigger the referral for psychological consultation. In other cases, the referral question arises in the course of medical assessment and treatment, e.g., a child admitted for chelation therapy of lead poisoning is noted to have a behavioral or developmental problem, or a child admitted for treatment of an infectious illness is noted to be excessively anxious.

Experienced consultants learn to look beyond the surface request to consider what may have motivated the referral. For example, requests for psychological consultation are often stimulated by child or parental behaviors that are confusing, upsetting, or threatening to the staff, e.g., a child who is noncompliant with treatment or parents who are angry about their child's care. Even when referrals are stimulated by complex interactional problems among staff, children, and their families, medical and nursing staff will often frame their referral questions in the language of psychological problems because they believe that this is the best way to obtain the psychologist's attention and response. For this reason, consultants need to be aware of contextual factors such as staff–family relationships that may influence the staff's appraisal of the child's problem and their reactions to the consultant's evaluation (Geist, 1977; Huszti & Walker, 1991). Each inpatient setting has a particular culture that reflects the technical demands of the clinical work, ages and developmental status of patients, and the attitudes of influential authorities, attending physicians, head nurses, senior residents, etc., toward psychological services.

In order to respond most effectively, consultants need to know what the physician (or nurse) expects from the consultation. Some requests are straightforward and discrete, e.g., a request to assess the developmental status of a young child with a history of prematurity. Others turn out to be more convoluted, time consuming, and highly charged. For example, a consultant might be asked to determine whether an adolescent with sickle cell anemia is "faking" his pain in order to manipulate the staff. Upon further questioning, the consultant learns that some of the nursing staff feel that the patient really doesn't need more pain medication but that the physician has a very different view. As this example suggests, unless the consultant clarifies the purpose of the assessment with referring staff, he or she can spend precious time addressing the "wrong" question. Even a brief discussion may help to clarify unrealistic or unusual expectations, e.g., a request that a behavioral management plan be implemented to "cure" a long-standing feeding disorder in a child who is expected to be hospitalized for several days. One of my all-time "favorite" unrealistic referral requests was for projective testing to reveal the affective world of an 8-month-old who was admitted for FTT. Whenever possible, a consultant should try to reshape or reframe such unrealistic referral requests into a more manageable form while addressing staff's underlying questions in some fashion.

A face-to-face or phone discussion can also clarify other key issues that will influence the consultation. For example, the length of time the child is expected to be in the hospital certainly influences the type of psychological service that can be provided. If the child is about to be discharged, it is preferable to arrange an outpatient assessment (if possible) rather than to try do a superficial, hurried assessment. On the other hand, consultation requests for children who are expected to have long hospital stays, e.g., a child undergoing extensive surgical procedures on a burn unit, often involve an expectation for a more extended commitment to provide help for the child or the staff.

Communicating with Multiple Staff

In pediatric teaching hospitals, multiple physicians are responsible for patient care. In some instances, overzealous and/or highly conscientious interns or residents may initiate psychological referrals without clearing them with the faculty, attending physicians, or community pediatricians who not only are legally responsible for the child's care but may have a long-standing relationship with the child and family. For this reason, psychological consultants should find out which physician is *primarily* responsible for the child's care to make sure that he or she is informed about the consultation and agrees that it is needed. This not merely a matter of courtesy but can make the difference between a successful and a problematic consultation.

Other professionals, such as those in nursing, child life, or social work, often have central roles in the child's care and hence are privy to important information about the child and his/her family that indicates a need for a psychological referral. In some instances, they will make referrals directly to psychology. Given such staff's access to children and families, it is clearly short-sighted to limit consultation requests to physicians. On the other hand, to avoid undermining the physician's authority and getting embroiled in staff disagreements about the need for a referral, the consultant should ensure that the primary physician is informed.

Informing the Child and Parents

It is also very important to find out from the referring physician whether the child and parents were informed about the request for psychological consultation, what they were told, and how they responded. Interns and residents order many procedures without necessarily informing children and their parents about each and every "routine" test. However, some physicians may manage psychological consultations the same way they handle procedures that are much less sensitive for the child and parents. Some physicians may also shy away from informing parents about the consultation because they don't want to offend them. In fact, some patients and their families may become upset when a psychologist is asked to assess or manage a problem, e.g., abdominal pain or chronic fatigue, that they have regarded as "physical" rather than psychological. Parents and children may feel threatened and/or offended that the staff feels the problem is "only in their head".

Because of such concerns, it is important to introduce oneself to the child and parents as a psychologist, clearly describe the reason for the consultation, and state what you intend to do, e.g., interview, observe, or conduct psychological testing. Such an introduction may sometimes unleash a torrent of feelings from parents who are stressed by the child's hospitalization and/or upset about their child's management. For example, in the course of consulting on cases of FTT where I was asked to assess the child's cognitive and emotional status and/or family factors that might be contributing to the problem, I was often confronted by parents who were confused and angered by the psychological consultation and, in some instances, their child's hospitalization. Some of these parents shared their concerns that staff felt that they were to blame for the child's problem and were not feeding their baby enough. Others were upset that the physicians had not been able to find a physical and hence treatable reason for their child's problem or concerned that there may be a physical cause that the physician had overlooked.

ACTIONS AND RESPONSIBILITIES IN PSYCHOLOGICAL CONSULTATION

Psychological consultation for hospitalized children tends to follow a traditional medical model in which the consultant's primary responsibilities involve assessment and communication to the physician about findings and advice concerning management (Freidson, 1970). The physician who requests a consultation retains primary responsibility for the patient and is under no obligation to follow the consultant's recommendations. In practice, however, many pediatric psychologists provide a wide range of clinical activities and interventions that go far beyond the basic consultation tasks.

Psychological Assessment

The varied methods of assessment used in psychological consultations on pediatric inpatient services depend greatly on the referral problems and time constraints (Drotar, 1977a; Huszti & Walker, 1991). Discrete, time-limited procedures such as administering a developmental test to a young infant are sufficient to address referral questions concerning cognitive assessment of infants' cognitive status. On the other hand, an adequate response to other referral questions, e.g., an request to evaluate a depressed child or a young child with a feeding disorder, will often require comprehensive, time-consuming assessment procedures, e.g., multiple interviews of child and family or repeated behavioral observations (Huszti & Walker, 1991).

In addition to psychological assessment procedures, consultants need to integrate information concerning the past medical history, current problems, and staff observations from the patient's chart. Although such comprehensive reviews of the child's past and current medical problems are time consuming, they can be extremely helpful. Because hospital staff tend to focus on the concrete, emergent problems of the moment, they may not appreciate the psychological meaning of key pieces of information concerning the child's family and/or medical history including important transitions in the course or trajectory of the child's condition (Strauss, Faberbaugh, Suczek, & Weiner, 1985). In this way, a psychological evaluation can provide the important function of integrating information from disparate sources into a coherent diagnostic picture and treatment plan. It is also very important to gather observations from other hospital staff who have contact with the child and his or her family because this will often reveal the "real story" behind the chart notes.

Communication to Staff

Communication of findings to hospital staff, which is a critical component of psychological consultation, is done by a note in the body of the chart or on a consultation sheet, or in both places. Such notes should be brief, factual, highly specific, and include three basic components: (1) a brief description of presenting problems, history, and procedures; (2) a brief appraisal of the child's problem; and (3) recommendations for management (Huszti & Walker, 1991). Moreover, it is often very helpful to supplement the chart note with a more detailed report for the referring physician and the child's medical record.

The following is an example of a chart note written for a 7-year-old child who was referred for psychological consultation during a hospitalization for diabetic ketoacidosis and diagnosis of insulin-dependent diabetes mellitus (IDDM). During the course of providing education for Johnny concerning his diabetes, various staff noted that he was quiet and withdrawn and questioned whether his level of language comprehension and expression was age-appropriate.

> The purpose of this assessment was to assess Johnny's level of intellectual ability and general comprehension. This was based on the Wechsler Intelligence Scale for Children, third edition. Consistent with the staff's observations, Johnny was cooperative

> with testing but very quiet and reserved. He did not initiate conversation and spoke only when spoken to. Moreover, his answers to questions were minimal.
>
> *Assessment*. Johnny's response to psychological testing indicated that he has a significant intellectual deficit. His Full-Scale IQ on the WISC III was 68, a performance that is in the range of mild mental retardation. Johnny's verbal abilities (IQ of 70) were comparable to his performance (nonverbal) skills (IQ of 70). However, there was some variation in his performance on individual tasks. Among verbal tasks, Johnny had the most difficulty with a task that reflected his comprehension of situations. In contract, he performed nearly at age level on a task that required him to copy marks according to a specific code.
>
> *Recommendations*. Johnny's intellectual deficits have several implications for his initial education and ongoing management of his diabetes. For example, explanations of his condition and treatment should correspond with his mental age (about 5 years) rather than his chronological age and should be repeated. It would be useful to also have Johnny repeat back concepts and instructions to ensure that he understands them. He would also benefit from concrete visual educational materials involving pictures rather than lengthy verbal explanations. Johnny's comprehension problems and shyness could make it difficult for him to describe symptoms and illness-related problems to family members and physicians. For this reason, it may be helpful to structure more frequent follow-up visits than is typical for children his age with diabetes. Finally, Johnny would benefit from a special class placement and a speech pathology evaluation.

As in other clinical situations (Seagull, 1979), the consultation note can help to advocate for the hospitalized child's needs, to modify staff's perceptions, e.g., helping them to see that an angry child might also be scared, and to educate staff concerning the contributions of psychological assessment and intervention. To accommodate to the staff's primary interest in the "bottom line" of management, recommendations should be both generous and specific.

Giving Direct Feedback to Staff

In addition to chart notes, which are the permanent record of the child's care, it is also important to provide direct feedback to staff by phone or, ideally, by face-to-face contact. Such feedback allows them to ask questions, register concerns, and make suggestions. Such communications are also needed to coordinate the disposition for a child and family, to discuss roles and responsibilities in the arrangement plan, and to clarify the plans for follow-up. One-to-one communication also can provide an excellent, albeit brief, opportunity for informal teaching.

Feedback to Parents and Child

Communication with medical, nursing, and other staff should not preclude the psychologist's talking with parents and/or the child concerning relevant findings and impressions from the assessment. Because it may be difficult for parents to ask for such feedback, let alone locate the psychologist in a busy hospital setting, psychologists need to take the initiative in giving feedback to families. In my experience, parents and children are most interested in answers to practical questions, e.g., what treatment or follow-up will be needed when my child returns home? How can we obtain necessary services? Will my child and I continue to see you?

Arranging Follow-Up

The consultant's role in management and follow-up of hospitalized children depends on the presenting problems, the results of the assessment, and practical considerations. In some cases, the consultant's communication of their results will be sufficient to allow the physician to conduct appropriate management. In other cases, the consultation may signal the beginning of intensive contact with the child for support and psychotherapy during the hospitalization and after the child returns home. The consultant's ongoing clinical responsibilities and the family's distance from the center may make psychological follow-up at the center unrealistic. For this reason, pediatric psychologists have to utilize considerable ingenuity in planning clinical interventions and supportive contact (Drotar *et al.*, 1982).

SPECIALIZED CONSULTATION PROCEDURES

Although a responsive, case-by-case consultation approach is a critical ingredient of assessment and clinical management, it does not address the complex system-related issues that influence the staff's appraisal of referral problems and management. (Geist, 1977; Mullins *et al.*, 1992). For example, the request for a psychological evaluation of a 3-year-old child, Chad, who had been hospitalized off and on for over a year as a result of short bowel syndrome, illustrated the complex role of staff-related conflict in management. Most of the nursing staff had become very attached to Chad during the course of his lengthy hospitalization. Serving in many ways as his surrogate parents, they had conflicting views about how to manage his behavior. Such disagreements became more intense when Chad began to assert his will, refuse his medication, and throw tantrums when he couldn't get his way. Some nursing staff felt that their colleagues were much too lenient with Chad, while others felt that their colleagues' expectations were too high. The overt request to me was to evaluate Chad's emotional status and help develop a plan for Chad's behavioral management. However, the implicit request was for me to validate some of the staff's concerns that their colleagues had "spoiled" Chad by giving in to him and created a "monster". Chad's management required coordination among several medical subspecialties, e.g., pediatrics, GI, and surgery, pediatric house staff who rotated on and off service each month, nursing staff, social work, occupational therapy, and child life. Chad's child life worker assumed a primary role in providing emotional support for him, while the social workers provided support to his mother, who had to cope with financial stresses and marital problems. However, no one consistently assumed responsibility for directing or coordinating his medical or psychological management. Consequently, one goal of this consultation involved helping the staff to coordinate a more consistent behavioral management plan for Chad.

STRUCTURING COLLABORATIVE CASE REVIEWS AND PLANNING

The problems of children such as Chad illustrate the need to develop consultation approaches that convene larger groups of staff to develop a working plan to manage salient problems (Huszti & Walker, 1991; Mullins *et al.*, 1992). This type of multidisciplinary case review has the following advantages over more traditional case-centered consultation: (1) comprehensive assessment based on observations from multiple staff, (2) promotion of more effective interdisciplinary problem solving concerning patient care, and (3) teaching about psychosocial management issues.

Implementing a Collaborative Case Review

To facilitate a case review, the psychologist-consultant (or whoever is leading and organizing the conference) needs to enlist the help of key staff, especially the head nurse and senior resident, to ensure the attendance of "key players" who have salient management roles. Planning a specific agenda that can be effectively accomplished in a limited time period (usually no more than an hour and in some cases less) is another key component of an effective case review. Prior discussion of the case with key staff will often reveal management issues and conflicts that will need to be considered.

In the first phase of a case review, the consultant discusses the general purpose of the meeting and specific goals. In the next phase of the case review, data gathering, one obtains the staff's observations concerning the specific problems that are of concern, the interventions they have tried, and their appraisal of their effectiveness. Because some participants will be more reticent (or outspoken) than others, the designated leader of the case review should ensure that participants have an opportunity to give their input.

The next phase of a case review, formulating a plan, requires considerable ingenuity because many of the problems that are brought to such meetings do not have clear or easy solutions. In order to be most effective, the staff needs to set priorities and come to some agreement on a plan, even if it is only a preliminary "working model". The goals and principles of a plan, e.g., to help the child demonstrate improved self-control, as well as specific recommendations, e.g., time-outs in response to tantrums, should be clearly stated.

Follow-Up

The final and in many ways most important phase of the case review meeting concerns implementation and follow-up. To help ensure that an agreed-upon plan is followed, the consultant should follow up with the persons who have accepted responsibility for implementing the plan. Putting what may look like even a very simple management plan in place can be very difficult, given the need to coordinate multiple staff. In some cases, it may be necessary if not critical to convene a subgroup of key staff to review how the plan is operating and to make necessary modifications. A follow-up meeting to review the child's progress, share additional concerns, and modify or add to the initial plan is often very useful. Follow-up case reviews are also an excellent place to acknowledge the time, energies, and interest of staff who have been involved in implementing a plan. Because staff may have different understandings about the plan of action, it is useful to document the plans that were discussed in the group meetings in the chart. Different staff members, e.g., nursing, pediatrics, child life, should be encouraged to contribute their own notes as well.

IMPLEMENTING ONGOING CASE REVIEWS

Collaborative case reviews on individual patients can be a very effective means of coordinating interdisciplinary planning concerning difficult problems. However, medical and nursing staff also have ongoing needs to coordinate care and learn about recurrent psychosocial issues that arise in patient care and behavioral management. Moreover, the problems of individual children and their families raise recurrent issues concerning patient care policy that require ongoing discussion and planning. Weekly psychosocial rounds modeled after the collaborative case review proved to be a useful forum to plan for a wide range of patient management issues on our adolescent division, a 25-bed acute care unit (Drotar, 1977b). Because the patient population included a large number of adolescents with serious illnesses, family reactions to chronic illness have been a consistent theme of the meetings, as shown in the following case vignette.

John, an 11-year-old boy with acute monocytic leukemia, experienced massive internal bleeding, had difficulty breathing, and was critically ill. He recently underwent a tracheotomy and, although he remained quite alert, could not communicate his feelings in words. Some nurses were quite concerned about what they perceived as the family's denial of the seriousness of John's condition. As time went on, the family's continuing presence became increasingly difficult for the staff. Feelings of tension erupted in arguments between the family and staff concerning John's care and visiting privileges for relatives.

The case review focused on gathering information and developing a consistent psychological approach to this family. John was the eldest son of parents who had been separated during most of his life. He had long been cared for by his mother, maternal grandmother, and aunt, who were of the Black Muslim faith. His grandmother had long been the dominant force in the family, which was quite close-knit and included a large number of relatives, all of whom wished to visit John because of his precarious physical condition. However, family members did not express their feelings to the staff.

Confused by the family's culture, many staff focused on the family's problems, particularly their "overprotectiveness." John's care had also engendered conflicts among the staff. Some of the African-American nurses felt that their Caucasian colleagues had been blinded by prejudice and had been unfair to the family by denying them unlimited visiting privileges.

Once these issues were aired, it was easier for the staff to coordinate a plan to support John and his family. John's primary physician agreed to take a more active role by talking with John and his family concerning his condition, confirming the fact that he was very sick. Because John had expressed great anxiety about hospital procedures such as tests and shots, the intern and nurses agreed to spend some time with John discussing the purpose and nature of the treatment procedures. The nursing staff recognized the family's sense of helplessness and tried to enhance their comfort in this setting. The head nurse discussed the policies concerning family participation with John's family, empathized with the family's recent emotional struggles, and asked them how they felt about the response of the staff to their family. The staff communicated their respect for the family's culture by offering John a special hospital tray in keeping with their religious and cultural preferences. In addition, the staff accommodated to the now constant presence of John's extended family. As they engaged in more frequent conversations with family members and learned more about them, the family's reactions became more understandable.

Liaison with Other Professional Staff

The presence of house staff who rotate on and off the unit, high turnover of nursing staff, and inconsistent support from attending physicians can limit the effectiveness of ongoing case review meetings. For this reason, coordinated efforts among many professional disciplines, e.g., nursing, child life, and social work, are necessary to share the work of preparation and leadership of the meetings, underscore the importance to the medical staff, and provide mutual support (see Chapter 5). In my experience, high levels of preparation and planning are required to develop and sustain successful ongoing meetings on hospital divisions. Such planning efforts also provide a way to take a "pulse" on unusual work demands that may affect the staff's participation and/or response to meetings.

Group Problem Solving to Enhance Policy and Practice

Ongoing case reviews can facilitate useful changes in ward policy, e.g., staffing, interprofessional communication, that facilitate management of psychosocial problems. For example, many of the patients who were hospitalized on our adolescent unit were young adults with cystic fibrosis (CF), some of whom were terminally ill. Patient deaths created extraordinary stresses for the families, the nurses and physicians, and other patients. Many of the patients with CF knew one another, sometimes very well. All of these factors generated helplessness and confusion among the staff about what to say to various patients and their families after a patient died. Perhaps as an attempt to bring order to such confusion, the division had developed an unwritten policy (the origins of which were obscure) to shut patients' doors immediately after a patient died. At several case review meetings, many staff expressed concerns that this policy was not helpful, as it intensified some patients' anxieties.

A working group consisting of the head nurse and some of her staff, me, child life, social work, and attending physicians was formed to discuss this policy and to consider other ways of interacting with patients and their families (Drotar & Doershuk, 1979). Eventually, we developed a more open policy of informing patients that there had been a death. At the point that patients were informed by the nursing staff, they were given the opportunity to discuss their feelings. In addition, the child life staff held meetings with small groups of interested patients to allow an additional opportunity for them to discuss their feelings about the death and/or other issues related to their hospitalization.

TEACHING THROUGH CASE REVIEWS

An interdisciplinary case discussion, which is a case review that is attended by multiple staff, is an excellent vehicle to integrate teaching and clinical management. However, this method requires the consultant to quickly generate useful clinical or research "pearls" that fit with the case discussion. For example, the staff's concerns about a child's reaction to a terminal illness can provide an opportunity for a brief discussion of research concerning the stages of children's understanding of death or parents' anticipatory grief and reactions to stress. Moreover, experienced consultants will often make ample use of clinical examples from their experience in order to help the staff generate options for clinical management, to think through the costs and benefits of different options, and to come to a reasonable decision (Caplan & Caplan, 1993). Effective consultant teachers are humble "experts" who give their teaching expertise freely but in such a way that it does not dominate their interactions with staff or undermine their confidence.

Ongoing case reviews can also identify staff needs for teaching. There is no shortage of potential topics for in-service presentations, e.g., parental grief, children's concepts of death, psychological development of children with chronic illness. Because the ideas and requests for teaching conferences will often outstrip the time, expertise, and interest of any one consultant, it is best to spread the work load by involving multiple professionals and speakers from the community.

Specialized teaching conferences can also be developed to address the management problems that are typically presented by children on different inpatient units. For example, in response to residents' interest in learning more about child development, we developed a teaching conference format of "live" demonstrations of developmental assessments on a 25-bed acute care division for infants up to age 2 years (Drotar & Malone, 1982). Based on discussion with the senior resident, cases were selected to illustrate particular clinical problem, e.g., FTT, mental retardation, or normal child development. In most but not all cases, children who were presented were observed and assessed prior to the conference. Following presentation of the child's history, the residents observed the child's response to developmental testing. This was accompanied by an explanation of the nature of test procedures, observations of the child's response to the testing, and evaluation of the child's intellectual strengths and deficits. The case conference format allowed the pediatric staff to check their own observations of children against the results of the assessment. Their observations served as a springboard for discussion of management of developmental problems. One useful byproduct of this teaching conference was more frequent and more appropriate referrals of children for psychological assessment.

5

Collaborating with Other Professions in Pediatric Settings

NEED FOR BROAD-BASED INTERDISCIPLINARY COLLABORATION

In order to thoroughly explicate specific professional issues, this book focuses on issues related to psychologists' collaborations with pediatricians. However, this emphasis should not be construed as a comment on the lack of importance of collaboration with other professionals. Although there are some settings, such as community practice, in which psychologists work only with pediatricians, most hospital-based psychological collaboration takes place in a multidisciplinary context (Mechanic, 1978). In most pediatric settings, psychologists are but one of many professions who provide comprehensive medical and psychological care to children and their families. The purpose of this chapter is to consider issues related to psychologists' collaboration with multiple professionals.

The overall impact of psychologists' efforts in pediatric settings depends on the quality of their collaboration with other professions for several reasons. One is that much of the care that is provided to patients and their families in inpatient and outpatient settings, especially for children with chronic conditions or complex psychosocial problems, is provided by other professions. In many settings, staff in social work, nursing, occupational and physical therapy, speech pathology, child life, etc. are assigned to individual inpatient divisions or to comprehensive care programs. Moreover, because they have contact with a large number of patients, such professionals are often privy to important psychological information, e.g., about the child's level of distress, parents' questions or concerns about a procedure, or family problems, that are not necessarily shared with the child's physician. For this reason, they are in a primary position to sensitize physicians to the psychological needs of children and their family. Moreover, in many pediatric settings, other professions provide the majority of "psychosocial" services. For example, nursing staff have primary day-to-day responsibilities to administer treatments to children and meet their needs for emotional support. Child life staff provide front-line resources to enhance emotional support and coping resources of hospitalized children (Thompson, 1989). Social workers provide family support and assessment of family problems and coordination of care and follow-up with community agencies. Over and beyond those professions that are traditionally identified with providing psychosocial services, a great many others such as speech pathology, occupational and physical therapy, respiratory therapy, etc. contribute to the quality of care that is provided to children and families in hospital settings. In view of the salience of these professionals' roles, pediatric psychologists should carefully consider how their work best complements rather than competes with that of their colleagues.

There are other compelling practical reasons to make proactive interdisciplinary planning an integral part of any pediatric psychology program. Compared with their pediatric colleagues, psychologists and their colleagues in social work, psychiatry, and child life are in the minority in most hospital settings. For this reason, cooperative interdisciplinary planning is necessary to advocate for and demonstrate the efficacy of psychosocial services. Moreover, a cooperative interdisciplinary relationship can be an important source of support. Psychologists and their colleagues in child life, social work, and psychiatry who work in pediatric settings for any length of time are stressed if not overwhelmed by the complexity, poignancy, and sheer volume of the psychosocial problems that they are called on to evaluate and solve. Many families who are referred for psychological services have difficult medical problems that are intertwined with extraordinary family and psychological problems, e.g., family disruption, parental emotional disturbances. All but the most naive (or arrogant) of pediatric psychologists eventually learn that they cannot possibly manage each and every one of the problems that are referred in their direction. Consequently, the professional expertise, direct help, and emotional support of other professions becomes critical to sustain a reasonable level of enthusiasm for clinical work as well as for professional stimulation and growth.

An alternative to collaborative interdisciplinary partnership is an isolated or competitive approach that is fueled by beliefs that one's profession is the most useful or effective. However, interprofessional competition or isolation results in several serious problems such as fragmented clinical care, duplication of services, and lack of efficient service (Friedman, 1985). Pediatricians and family members may have difficulty effectively using services that are not well coordinated. Many pediatricians find the overlap in the roles of psychologists, social workers, and child psychologists to be confusing, even if these services are relatively well coordinated.

Difficult and compelling clinical problems seen in pediatric settings, e.g., suicidal behavior, child abuse and neglect, generate a great deal of anxiety and concern among pediatric colleagues, especially among inexperienced staff and residents, that may intensify confusion concerning professional roles. For example, initially in our setting, it was not uncommon for pediatric residents to issue a set of multiple requests for consultation from psychology, social work, and psychiatry on the same patients, especially those with disturbing problems, e.g., suicidal adolescents. This practice was not only inefficient but very confusing to families.

OBSTACLES TO INTERDISCIPLINARY COLLABORATION

Administrative Organization

Although close interprofessional collaboration may be in the best interests of children and families, it is very difficult to accomplish in many pediatric hospitals, partly because of the separate administrative organization of individual professions (Friedman, 1985). Each profession has its own lines of authority, set of responsibilities, and professional standards of care. Such separate organizational structures help to develop and sustain professional identify and support, which are certainly necessary in medical settings. On the other hand, they may interfere with planning and implementing interdisciplinary programs for various patient groups. For example, many populations, especially children with chronic illness, who are seen in great numbers in pediatric settings, optimally require comprehensive care that is provided by different professionals (Sabbeth & Stein, 1990). However, interdisciplinary care is very difficult to organize , plan, and implement, partly because each professional group has separate professional priorities and incentive structures.

Turf, Territory, and Competition

The separate administrative organization characteristics of professional functioning in hospital settings also can contribute to interprofessional competition, especially when there are limited resources, e.g., space and funds for salaries (Glenn, 1987). Elfant (1985) eloquently captured this feature in his stark description of hospitals as: "onerous city states where different classes uneasily coexist . . . territory is coveted and protected, and insidious rivalries abound . . ." (p. 57). In my experience, it is not uncommon for those who work in hospital settings to be quite protective of what they regard as their professional turf. There can be a fine line between professional pride, which is an admirable characteristic, and what Sarason (1972) calls "preciousness", defined as the belief that one's profession is uniquely equipped to perform a task or solve a problem, which is a less admirable attribute.

Although a strong sense of professional preciousness is not only unrealistic but divisive, most of us fall prey to its spell. As a new psychologist in a pediatric hospital, I must admit to having strong feelings of competitiveness with the child psychiatry service that already had a part-time presence in this, or should I say *my* setting. Being possessive of what I saw as "my territory", I wanted to make sure that pediatricians appreciated the unique advantages of a psychologist's professional role and contributions. As it turned out, I soon had more than enough to do, and my sensitivities about pediatricians' utilization of child psychiatry consultation turned out to be unfounded and among the least of my problems (Drotar, 1976).

As this example shows, professionals in pediatric settings tend to be protective of the services that they have developed and plan to develop. They may feel threatened and feel criticized by consultants from other disciplines who have a "better idea" about how such services should be organized and delivered. Such a threat may reflect the difficulty of establishing a professional beachhead in pediatric settings. On the other hand, to ensure long-term professional growth and survival in pediatric settings, there are certainly advantages to a "strength in numbers" concept that relies on coalition building among different professions in areas of mutual concern.

Differences in Professional Cultures

In one sense, nonphysicians who work together on teaching, research, and service programs in pediatric settings collaborate on the "neutral" turf of hospital culture. However, interprofessional behavior is shaped by professional values, ethics, and practice standards that have been strongly inculcated in profession-specific patterns of training and practice (Katon & Kleinman, 1981). Based on their training, different professional groups tend to set discrepant priorities for clinical assessment and intervention with pediatric populations. For example, many social workers often have more of a family- or parent-centered focus to their work than many psychologists, psychiatrists, or pediatricians. Child psychiatrists have more experience with children with severe psychopathology and medication management than psychologists with behavioral management. Various professionals use different languages to describe, report, and communicate about their work and may have different concepts about diagnoses and interventions (Hamlett & Stabler, in press). For example, physicians are trained to make a differential diagnosis in order to recommend a treatment plan, whereas psychologists are much more comfortable with a functional approach to assessment and treatment planning that emphasizes a description of the child's behavioral and developmental competencies and deficits. Different professions also place discrepant values on the importance of research in guiding practice (Drotar & Sturm, in press).

Because the differences in professional language, concepts, and practice that heighten tensions in interdisciplinary collaboration are deeply rooted in years of training and practice, they do not yield to easy reconciliation. At the very least, interprofessional differences in patterns of practice may interfere with understanding, communication, and conjoint planning. Moreover, to the extent that an individual considers his or her particular profession as having the sole or primary claim as the "only" and right clinical viewpoint, interprofessional conflicts become more serious.

Professional Roles and Boundaries

In my experience, individuals from different professions who work together in clinical, teaching, and research activities may find that their roles become more interchangeable. For example, psychologists who work with social workers may find that they adopt a family-centered perspective that involves work with parents; social workers may come to utilize behavioral methods in their clinical work. Such "crossing over" of traditional professional roles and boundaries can be very stimulating because of the opportunity to learn a different perspective and practice different skills. On the other hand, such blurring of roles can also be threatening and anxiety provoking. If a member of another profession can carry out some of our work, we may see ourselves as less special (Sarason, 1972). Because interprofessional roles are not completely interchangeable, the "rules" for sharing of roles and responsibilities among different professions must be worked out in practice. Moreover, individuals may have different thresholds for what they regard as an infringement on their professional roles (see Chapter 9).

ENHANCING INTERDISCIPLINARY COLLABORATION

Commitment to Interdisciplinary Cooperation

How can a pediatric psychologist develop and maintain effective interdisciplinary alliances while developing profession-specific collaborative relationships with pediatricians? In order to accomplish this admittedly difficult feat, one needs to adopt several basic assumptions. Perhaps the most important is the need to accept, value, and respect the contributions of one's colleagues in other professions. Such respect is not automatically or easily achieved but may be enhanced by training programs or on-the-job experiences that emphasize interdisciplinary contact and cooperation.

Commitment to an ecological perspective, i.e., that the psychological interests of children and families are best served by coherent organization of medical psychosocial care that is provided by each profession will also enhance interdisciplinary collaboration (Mullins *et al.*, 1992). In this model, the "whole" of the contributions made by multiple professions is seen as much greater than any of the "parts" that can be provided by any single profession.

Strategies that facilitate effective interdisciplinary collaboration are quite comparable to those that are useful in working with pediatricians. For example, psychologists who are visible, accessible, and useful to other professional staff will generally be utilized by them. Similar to work with pediatricians, consultation with other professions should be approached in a way that respects their competence and is sensitive to the threats that others may experience (Stabler, 1988). For this reason, psychologists who are new to a setting should endeavor to take careful and complete inventory of existing patterns of services in order to set work priorities that enhance rather than disrupt ongoing interdisciplinary collaboration.

Experienced staff also have valuable perspectives to contribute to new consultants concerning patterns of care and effective strategies. As a brand new psychologist fresh from postdoctoral training, I had many ideas about consultation, not all of which were realistic in my new setting. To help guide my efforts, I sought out and relied on the advice of senior social workers and nursing staff concerning the needs and priorities for services and information about programs that had been developed and unsuccessful strategies. Such information was critical to avoid reinventing services and threatening colleagues.

Collaborative Program Development

Interdisciplinary collaboration is generally more effective when one truly needs help and support from others and there is mutual opportunity to shape a new program. However, irrespective of whether one is developing a program from scratch or trying to influence a well-established one, it is important to develop and implement one's goals by working closely with other professions. Strong interdisciplinary collaborative partnerships with social work and nursing were especially critical to the development of my own work. For example, I worked with social workers such as Mary Ann Ganofsky on an inpatient unit and chronic illness consultation (see Chapters 4 and 6). Moreover, my work with head nurses on the inpatient units and nurse practitioners in primary care, many of whom were providing ongoing care to children with chronic conditions, was invaluable (Drotar, Crawford, & Ganofsky, 1984).

Building Support for Interdisciplinary Collaboration

One useful antidote to isolation and competition among consultants in a pediatric setting is the development of regular forums for interdisciplinary communication (see Chapter 4 for descriptions of specific methods such as the collaborative case review). At the very least, such forums involve regular discussions of shared cases. More frequent and formal structures for case discussion and collaboration may be needed when many professions are providing services to similar populations (Drotar & Ganofsky, 1976). Successful collaboration will often facilitate the development of additional structures to enhance interdisciplinary communication. For example, in my setting, successful clinical collaboration among psychology, nursing, social service, and child life led to the development of interdisciplinary case conferences for staff and trainees in which we presented clinical cases and discussed strategies of managing difficult clinical and consultation problems (Drotar, 1977a).

Nonphysicians who consult to pediatricians in medical settings often share common frustrations, which can help to forge a common bond and mutual support. I have also found it very helpful to involve other professions in training psychologists in consultation. Psychology trainees can benefit from observing social workers, speech pathologists, child life workers, etc. in their work with children and their families. Familiarizing psychology trainees with the contributions of other professions sensitizes them to the need for and importance of consultation with others. Such contact also has the considerable advantage of creating empathy for the professional work of other disciplines. One of the most useful experiences in my own clinical training was the opportunity to participate in an interdisciplinary team for the assessment of children with physical and developmental disabilities.

Managing Problems That Arise in Interdisciplinary Collaboration

As with physicians, collaboration with other professions does not always run smoothly. Several examples from my own experience illustrate the types of problems that can arise. For example, my chart notes from my assessment of a child with developmental problems troubled the speech pathologist who was assigned to the same division. She objected to my using descriptions of the child's expressive and receptive language to describe the child's cognitive functioning because she felt pediatricians could construe this note as substituting for a speech evaluation. I assured her that this was not my intention. Moreover, I addressed her concern by modifying my future chart notes.

Another issue arose in the course of our implementing research concerning the evaluation of a program of home-based intervention with children who were hospitalized for FTT and their families. This project was designed to evaluate the efficacy of a new outreach program that complemented rather than replaced existing care. To implement the study, our research staff of social workers, nurses, and child development specialists contacted families during the child's hospitalization for FTT. However, our presence was confusing and at times threatening to hospital staff who interacted with the same families. Our staff made many presentations to nursing, pediatric, and social work staff explaining the goals of the program and communicating our strong interest in working together. Once the staff recognized that our intentions were not to replace but to complement their services and that they could reduce their work loads by referring families to us, our work became less threatening.

FUTURE NEEDS

One of the most important but neglected issues in pediatric psychologists' writings on collaboration and consultation is the issue of collaboration with other disciplines. I have the impression that much more of such work actually transpires than is written about (see Schroeder's work on collaborative practice in Chapter 3 or Kazak and Beele's description of their psychosocial service program for children with cancer in Chapter 6). One important future task is for pediatric psychologists to describe their collaborations with other professions in greater depth, including the special issues and problems that arise. Moreover, data concerning the nature and efficacy of interdisciplinary collaboration in specialized programs, e.g., for children with chronic illness, would be particularly instructive (see Chapter 6).

6

Collaboration in Programs for Children with Chronic Health Conditions and Their Families

Collaborative clinical care and research programs appear to be especially important for certain pediatric populations. Children with chronic physical conditions are one such group. The extraordinary stressors related to the management and treatment of chronic physical illness and handicap and concomitant risk for mental health problems for children (Gortmaker & Sappenfield, 1984) and psychological distress for parents (Wallander, Varni, Babani, & Wilcox, 1989) create a need to develop effective ways of providing support to affected families and their children. Development and implementation of such programs often require a high level of collaboration among pediatricians, psychologists, and other professions. The purpose of this chapter is to discuss the issues involved in such collaborative teaching and clinical programs.

BARRIERS TO COLLABORATIVE COMPREHENSIVE CARE

Despite compelling reasons to integrate mental health services with the medical care of children with chronic conditions and their families (Drotar & Bush, 1985), significant barriers often interfere with the development of collaborative comprehensive care programs (Sabbeth & Stein, 1990). Physicians who provide ongoing medical care for children with chronic physical problems may not use psychological services for several reasons: reluctance to label their patients as having a mental health problem for fear this would stress the family; uncertainty about behavioral or mental health norms for children with chronic conditions; or primary focus on the child's medical needs (Sabbeth & Stein, 1990). Moreover, the experience of providing care to children with chronic conditions and their families departs significantly from the acute care model that dominates medicine. The management of chronic and lifethreatening physical problems not only generates difficult emotional reactions in physicians and other professional caregivers (Artiss & Levine, 1973) but requires special skills in communication, coordination of care, anticipatory guidance, and treatment planning that are not emphasized in traditional medical training (Daeschner & Cerreto, 1985; Grose & Goodrich, 1985).

Even if their psychological problems are recognized by a pediatrician, some children may not receive necessary mental health services because of practical obstacles such as financial costs of care, limitations in physical functioning as a result of the medical condition, and lack of available services and/or trained professionals in the community (Sabbeth & Stein, 1990).

The necessity to develop collaborative comprehensive care for children with chronic physical and/or developmental problems transcends the need to integrate mental health services with medical care. Children with chronic physical problems often have complex medical needs and treatments that may need to be modified depending on the course of their illness. The problems of many children with chronic conditions involve multiple organ systems and hence necessitate the efforts of multiple medical specialties. Others need a wide range of interventions, e.g., physical therapy, speech therapy, or, in the case of technology-dependent children, home-based care, all of which involve many professionals.

The diagnosis and treatment of children with chronic physical problems creates many difficult decisions concerning timing and priorities for treatment and sharing of professional responsibility (Artiss & Levine, 1973; Kanthor, Pless, Satterwhite, & Myers, 1974). Professional staff may have very different philosophies about the value and necessity for children and family members to participate in decisions that relate to their medical and physical care. Unless these professionals have a way to communicate with one another and organize their feedback to the family, parents and children may experience their efforts as confusing if not overwhelming (Klerman, 1985). At its best, interdisciplinary comprehensive care provides a vehicle to help organize, structure, and improve the level of communication and decision making among various professionals as well as between parents and professionals.

Despite widespread professional recognition of the need for comprehensive care for children with chronic physical and/or developmental problems, such programs are very difficult to develop and sustain for several reasons. Comprehensive care involves the kind of support, advocacy, and planning services that are difficult to support financially. Comprehensive care also requires meshing of different professional perspectives concerning clinical care, language, and perceived priorities for services (Drotar & Sturm, in press). The fact that one has achieved success in his or her particular profession by no means guarantees that he or she will function effectively in a comprehensive care team.

DEVELOPING MODELS OF COLLABORATIVE COMPREHENSIVE CARE

In many settings, the availability of medical care for children with chronic conditions is well in place before the need for collaborative comprehensive care programs is "discovered" by staff who must manage very troubling psychological and ethical problems that are raised (Perrin, 1992). Consequently, in many settings, collaborative comprehensive care programs evolve gradually in response to emerging needs.

Koocher, Sourkes, and Keane (1979) presented an instructive description of the development of comprehensive care consultation in pediatric oncology at the Sidney Farber Cancer Institute in Boston. Initially, psychological consultation was provided to the oncology unit in this setting only on an emergency basis. This model resulted in little follow-up, minimal staff support, crisis-oriented management of psychological problems, and a nonpreventive approach to management. Koocher and his colleagues' interests in expanding the case-focused consultation in to a more comprehensive approach meshed well with those of the nursing staff, who requested that they be available to them on a consistent, routinely scheduled basis. This expanded time commitment eventually led to improved referral practices, the development of weekly psychosocial rounds on the unit, and a comprehensive approach whereby the psychology team worked with a large number of families (patients, siblings, parents, and extended families are seen) on inpatient and outpatient units (Koocher *et al.*, 1979). Over time, this program developed a range of services in which some patients, such as those with bone cancer, were seen from the time of diagnosis, and others were referred by medical, social work, or nursing staff at any point during their illness. Interdisciplinary collaboration was enhanced by offering in-service training on such topics as psychological aspects of childhood cancer and intervention strategies. Not surprisingly, this level of collaborative work proved to be time consuming, as each of the half-time psychological consultants typically spent more than 20 hours per week in direct service, supervision, teaching rounds, and consultation with medical and nursing staff on case management.

The above description illustrates how shared clinical experiences can facilitate deepening professional commitment and specialized services for children with chronic conditions. One salient advantage of such sustained collaboration is the development of specialized management that is tailored to specific medical and psychological issues that are encountered with various populations.

Collaborative Team Functioning

In order to sustain the staff availability and planning that are the hallmarks of comprehensive care, professionals need to develop ways to share information, make decisions, plan interventions, and support one another. In a comprehensive care program, team members share responsibility for the planning and timing of medical and psychosocial interventions. Because more than one team member is usually involved with a given family, careful structuring of roles is required. Regular meetings provide a vehicle for team members to argue, question, and share their concerns about working with different families. Collaborators also can benefit from formal and informal means of mutual support to help manage their emotional reactions.

Shared responsibility for patient care usually involves some overlap in team members' roles. For example, each and every team member will develop the capacity to listen to the child's and parents' reactions and provide information concerning treatment and emotional support. In this way, children and family members have the benefit of contact with a network of professionals who are sensitive to their concerns. At the same time, the roles of different disciplines must be clearly delineated to avoid confusing families.

The high level of cooperation and interchangeability of professional roles that is characteristic of some collaborative comprehensive care teams can reflect a long history of working together in various collaborative trials by fire. In this regard, our experience in developing a comprehensive care program for children with end-stage renal failure is instructive, (Drotar, 1975; Drotar & Ganofsky, 1976; Drotar, Ganofsky, & Makker, 1979). At the time that we began this work in the mid-1970s, the technology of dialysis and transplantation had only recently become available for children and adolescents with end-stage renal failure at our hospital. However, the number of available kidneys was quite limited, and the possibility of chronic dialysis was uncertain. The first dialysis and transplantation program in our setting involved adults. However, several pediatric patients were deemed eligible, and pediatric nephrology began to provide care for them. Shortly after the program began, psychology, child psychiatry, and social work were requested to assess the psychological status of children, adolescents, and their families to determine their "suitability" as candidates for transplantation. We were very uncomfortable about conducting these assessments because we knew that our ability to predict which children and families would do well or poorly following a transplant was limited. As a group, we were clearly in uncharted clinical terrain.

As the numbers of children who were referred by us began to increase, Mary Ann Ganofsky, a social worker, and Suddesh Makker, a pediatric nephrologist, and I began to discuss the difficult clinical management and ethical issues raised by this group of children. We eventually decided to make a commitment to providing comprehensive care for *all* children and families who were referred to us. In retrospect, our strong collegial bonds were partly enhanced by the uncertainties and difficulties of this new technology and treatment. As we continued to work together, our collaboration evolved into mutual respect and close personal and professional relationships. Eventually, this work led to collaborative presentations and written descriptions of our work. Together, we developed a model of collaborative preventive intervention that had the following goals: (1) mastery of potentially disruptive anxiety related to the disease and its physical management; (2) a reasonable understanding of and adherence to necessary medical regimens; (3) integration of illness into family life, especially the reconciliation of family needs with those of the ill child; and (4) adaptation to hospital, school, and peers (Drotar & Ganofsky, 1976; Drotar *et al.*, 1984)

One key component of this model of care was continuous availability of the professional staff so that children and families were not abandoned at any point in the course of the illness and had a familiar person to turn to in times of crisis and with whom to share moments of triumph over illness-related adversity. Advocacy, defined as the use of professional knowledge of the child's illness, medical status, and treatments to intervene with agencies and professionals on behalf of the family, was another critical ingredient of preventive intervention.

Tensions and Stresses in Collaborative Care

Collaborative comprehensive care is not without its tensions. In our work, we disagreed about clinical management issues and were often stressed by the exposure to the insoluble medical and family problems experienced by a group of children with chronic, sometimes life-threatening conditions. We decided to divide up the clinical work on the basis of interest rather than along traditional professional lines. In some instances, my social work colleague, Ganofsky, provided some individual counseling to children with my consultation. In some instances, I saw parents, siblings, and other family members to give our team another perspective about difficult decisions concerning dialysis versus transplantation or family donors of a kidney.

Professionals in specialized comprehensive care programs typically find themselves immersed in special medical/ethical issues associated with the care of children with chronic conditions (Weithorn & McCabe, 1988). For example, psychologists may be asked to contribute their professional opinions concerning children's competence to consent to medical treatment (Schowalter, Ferholt, & Mann, 1973) or to participate in staff decisions concerning the costs and benefits of extraordinary treatments such as bone marrow transplantation or organ donation (Weithorn & McCabe, 1988). Such professional involvement is clearly not an integral part of typical clinical psychological training. Consequently, pediatric psychologists need to familiarize themselves with the nature of these ethical issues, their potential impact on children, families, and staff, as well as relevant research (Weithorn & Campbell, 1982).

In my experience, the stresses that surround ethical issues concerning the care of children with chronic, life-threatening conditions such as cancer can have a profound influence on professional staff, children, and families who find themselves inextricably involved in a series of very difficult interactions surrounding treatment decisions (Koocher, 1980). In our work with children with end-stage renal failure and their families, we found ourselves immersed in many such questions: Would prolonging children's lives with dialysis and transplantation reduce their quality of life? How should we best involve parents and siblings in decisions? Our personal and professional concerns with such ethical issues often dominated our team meetings. In response to these problems, we eventually developed a strong team commitment to shared decision making with children and families (Drotar *et al.*, 1982).

COLLABORATIVE MANAGEMENT OF CHRONIC PSYCHOPHYSIOLOGICAL PROBLEMS

Another group of children with chronic problems that challenge collaborative management are those with psychophysiological symptoms, e.g., failure to thrive (FTT), chronic pain, encopresis. A wide range of common problems fall into this category, including somatization or somatoform disorders (Routh, Ernst, & Harper, 1988). In contrast to many infectious diseases that are reliably recognized and have relatively specific, effective treatments, the diagnosis and treatment of psychophysiological disorders is more ambiguous and requires practitioners to address psychological and family influences during all phases of care (Engel, 1977). Moreover, the management of such problems involves very demanding communication with family members whose concepts of the etiology and management may differ dramatically from those of professionals (Drotar & Sturm, 1988).

Obstacles to Collaborative Management

Because many chronic psychophysiological problems require the physician and psychologist to play conjoint and active roles in clinical management and communication with the child and family, they raise special challenges for interprofessional collaboration. In some instances, physicians' frustrations concerning the ambiguity of symptoms, the lack of definitive interventions, and difficulty of working with families may lead to maladaptive approaches such as devaluing of the child's problem. For example, the child with a psychosomatic symptom may be seen as a "turkey," as having a problem that is "not physical," and as competing with children who are "really sick" for precious bed space. In some instances, once some physicians determine to their own satisfaction that the child's problem is primarily "psychological," they may reduce their level of clinical involvement and try to transfer the management of the child's care to the psychologist or another mental health professional. However, many children with chronic physical symptoms have problems that require ongoing clinical monitoring and treatment. Moreover, many of these children and parents still feel that their symptoms require the physician's involvement and may feel abandoned if their case is transferred to another professional.

The problems that can arise in the management of children with chronic somatic symptoms are shown in the following case illustration. An 8-year-old child presented with seizures that did not correspond to any known organic pathology but, nonetheless, were quite debilitating, resulting in many missed days of school. Psychological evaluation indicated that the child was coping with a number of severe family stresses, including the parents' fighting at home, and was very close to her mother. Moreover, the child's mother was very involved in closely monitoring and possibly reinforcing the child's symptoms. During the hospitalization, multiple clinical observations of the child's symptoms revealed that they did not correspond to any known pattern of seizures. Repeated EEGs were normal. Increasingly convinced that the child's symptoms reflected psychological rather than medical problems, the pediatrician and neurologist became much less involved with the child and family. The psychologists' attempts to engage the family in assessment counseling were met with a wall of resistance and insistence that the child was "not crazy". The parents then signed their child out against medical advice.

Collaborative Management of Chronic Psychophysiological Problems

To prevent negative outcomes as in the above case, collaborative integration of medical and psychological care is needed in the management of chronic physical problems such as FTT (Frank & Drotar, 1994), gastrointestinal disorders (Whithead & Schuster, 1985), and pain-related problems (McGrath, 1990; see Chapter 13). Collaborative programs have several important advantages over general services. First, psychological services can be introduced very early in the child's management and closely integrated into an overall plan for diagnosis and management. This approach gives the clear message to the child and family that psychological factors are important in clinical management and reduces the stigma that children and family members might experience about seeing a psychologist. Moreover, the close integration of the psychologist and pediatrician's work encourages the development of collaborative clinical management that address the child's physical and psychological problems in the same plan. In my experience, such management generally enhances communication with family members concerning the etiology and treatment of the child's symptoms. Consequently, children and families experience more support from the treatment team. Finally, collaborative management provides greater mutual professional support than is feasible in typical patterns of care.

PROGRAM DEVELOPMENT

The close interdisciplinary collaboration that is involved in the comprehensive care of children with chronic physical illness can facilitate the development of a multifaceted integrated program that includes teaching, research, and clinical services. However, in my experience it is very difficult to develop and sustain such comprehensive programs of service, teaching, and research in pediatric hospitals because of fiscal pressures, difficulties of sustaining continuity in professional staff, and the considerable emotional demands that are involved in such work.

One current example of what can be accomplished with such collaborative programs is the psychosocial services program that has been developed by Anne Kazak and her colleagues (Kazak & Beele, 1993) in the Division of Oncology at the Children's Hospital of Philadelphia (CHOP).

The purpose of this program is to provide comprehensive mental health services for children with cancer and their families and to conduct research related to the adjustment of this patient population. Based within a large pediatric oncology center in a university-affiliated children's hospital, the psychosocial services team consists of 12 full time staff members: four Ph.D. psychologists, six master's-level social workers, and two child life specialists. Additional staff include graduate-level trainees in clinical and school psychology and social work. This program provides a range of clinical services, teaching, and research that are funded in a variety of ways. For example, a Child Health Improvement Project (MCHIP) award supports two full-time staff members, portions of other psychosocial salaries, and other programs. The overall focus of the grant is the development of family-centered, community-based psychosocial and psychoeducational services for children with serious health care conditions. Research is funded by several grants from the National Cancer Institute.

Clinical Services: Example from the Program at CHOP

A wide range of clinical services are offered as a part of Kazak and Beele's (1993) program at CHOP. These include the following.

Primary Psychosocial Care. Every newly diagnosed child with cancer is assigned a member of the psychosocial staff who joins the patient's primary treatment team. A social worker or psychologist conducts an initial psychosocial evaluation of the child and family and provides support during the diagnostic workup and communication of diagnosis and treatment to the child and family. The primary psychosocial staff member assigned to a child and family continues to work with the family over the course of the child's inpatient or outpatient treatment.

Resources and Community Linkages. This program is closely linked with additional social, psychological, supportive, or financial services that are available in the community. Programs such as a school reintegration program have been developed to help promote family adjustment. Social security and the programs of the American Cancer Society are community resources that are often utilized. A handbook that describes programs and resources that are available to families is given to newly diagnosed families and is also made available on the inpatient unit.

Psychological Consultation. Patients can be referred to psychology staff for concerns about severe or chronic behavioral, emotional, or family problems at any point in the course of treatment or follow-up. Individual and family psychotherapy are provided as needed.

Support and Parent Education Groups. A weekly parents' group is open to all parents of children with cancer. A support group for parents of children with brain tumors meets once a month in the evening. A parent education and support group is available to parents twice a month in the outpatient clinic and is also open to parents of children on the inpatient unit.

Parent-to-Parent Support Network. Funded in part by the MCHIP grant, the Parent-to-Parent Support Network provides peer support for parents of newly diagnosed patients. "Support" parents are identified through referrals from staff, are at least 1 year out from diagnosis, and are perceived as coping well. These parents participate in an 18-hour training program in general counseling skills. Parents of newly diagnosed patients are then paired with the support parents. This program has recently been expanded to include consultation with staff at community sites.

Straight Talk About Recovering Teens (START). By providing friendship and encouragement, 15- to 24-year-old cancer survivors are helped to serve as positive role models and help newly diagnosed patients develop their own methods of coping.

For Brothers and Sisters Only. Siblings of patients have participated in 1-day workshops about childhood cancer conducted three times a year. Workshop activities have included medical education and play, videotapes, discussion, and recreational activities that promote the expression of feelings and enhancement of coping strategies.

Child Life Programs. A full-time child life specialist provides daily programming for outpatients within one area devoted to child play and other areas throughout the clinic (e.g., day hospital, procedure rooms). In addition, a large volunteer network has supplemented staffing on a daily basis and allowed for the expansion of small-group and individual activities. The inpatient child life program has been a well established part of the hospital program. A full-time child life specialist provides therapeutic programming in the playroom and support to patients who are confined to their hospital rooms.

Educational Liaison/School Consultation. For the past 15 years, an annual day-long program for patients, teachers, other school personnel, and patients' siblings has been held at CHOP. This program typically consists of two panel discussions (patients, parents and educations), a keynote address, and about 10 workshops addressing specific issues (e.g., learning problems, cancer in children at different developmental stages). A series of smaller educational programs (e.g., on parent advocacy) have also been provided. In the school reintegration program, nurses and psychosocial staff are available to visit schools, talk with school personnel, and provide age-appropriate presentations for patients' classmates.

Psychological Evaluation. Psychological evaluations and school consultations have been provided for patients experiencing learning difficulties or concerns regarding appropriate educational placement. This program places a strong emphasis on helping parents advocate for their children within their educational system and promoting collaborative relationships between families and schools.

Neuropsychological testing has also been provided regularly. Several distinct groups of patients have been targeted for evaluations before radiation begins. In addition, prospective data on the effects of current radiation are gathered in several protocols. These include (1) those with relapsed leukemia who will receive cranial irradiation, (2) children referred to bone marrow transplant (with and without total-body irradiation), and (3) newly diagnosed patients who will receive cranial irradiation.

Communication with Other Staff. Two psychosocial rounds are held weekly, one with the oncology attending and inpatient medical staff and another with the inpatient nursing staff. Psychosocial staff attend other rounds as needed and participate in family meetings and patient management conferences. Psychosocial staff rotate responsibility for editing the *PsychoSocial Services Times!* (*PSST!*), a newsletter that is circulated three or four times a year with information about psychosocial activities and other articles of interest to oncology staff.

Psychosocial staff also collaborate closely with programs that are based outside the Division of Oncology. As an example, the Bereavement Program in the Home Care Department offers services to oncology patients while psychosocial staff collaborate with bereavement program staff.

Research

Research concerning a wide range of psychosocial issues related to childhood cancer is an integral part of this program (Kazak, 1993; Kazak & Nachman, 1991). Active projects include the following.

Analgesia Protocol for Procedures in Oncology. The goals of this study include the development of an integrated psychological/pharmacological protocol for children with cancer having invasive procedures, expanding education and interventions for children and their parents around distressing procedures, preparing programs and materials for staff education, and using quantitative methods to assess the efficacy of the intervention program. Specific research projects within the analgesia protocol for procedures in oncology (APPO) include (1) a cross-sectional study of 70 patients with leukemia and their parents, conducted prior to the initiation of APPO (Kazak, Blackall, Boyer, Brophy, Daller, & Himelstein, 1994a); (2) a prospective study comparing pharmacological and preventive behavioral intervention with pharmacological treatment alone; (3) an analysis of videotape data utilizing behavioral rating systems; and (4) prospective assessment of the impact of introducing change on staff in a complex pediatric setting (Kazak, Boyer, Brophy, Johnson, Schear, Covelman, & Scott, 1994b).

Stress, Support, Survival: Children at Medical Risk. This collaborative study with the University of California at Los Angeles focuses on the risk and protective factors associated with more and less adaptive psychological functioning in children and their parents who have ended treatment. Based on a social–ecological model of serious childhood illness (Kazak, 1989; Kazak & Meadows, 1989), a pilot study of 64 patients who had leukemia and their parents demonstrated the utility of a posttraumatic stress model for understanding the types of ongoing difficulties experienced by some survivors and their parents (Kazak, Stuber, Gorchinsky, Houskamp, Christakis, & Fasiraj, 1992).

FUTURE NEEDS

In collaboration with their colleagues, pediatric psychologists have developed an impressive and ever-expanding repertoire of specialized knowledge concerning the management of children with chronic health conditions. Interested readers should consult the following edited volumes: Gross and Drabman (1990), Magrab (1978a,b), Olson, Mullins, Gillman, and Chaney (1994), Routh (1988), and Russo and Varni (1982). To build on this impressive body of work, there is a continuing need to document the efficacy of psychological interventions including comprehensive care for children with chronic health conditions. Several promising interventions have been reported. For example, Delameter, Bubb, Davis, Smith, Schmidt, White, and Santiago (1990) found that children with insulin-dependent diabetes mellitus (IDDM) who received family-based self-management training, which involved helping patients to utilize self-monitoring of blood glucose in the first few months after diagnosis, had better levels of metabolic control 2 years after diagnosis than patients treated conventionally.

In another innovative study, Varni, Katz, Colegrove, and Dolgin (1993) documented the effectiveness of an innovative social skills training program on the psychological and social support of children with newly diagnosed cancer. Children who received a structured curriculum involving social cognitive problem solving, assertive training, and handling teasing and name calling that was taught through modeling, behavioral rehearsal, and corrective feedback demonstrated fewer behavioral problems and greater classmate and teacher support at 9-month follow-up than a group who received a school reintegration intervention without social skills training. Finally, in an impressive follow-up study, Stein and her colleagues have described the positive impact of family-centered home-based comprehensive care on the long-term emotional adjustment of children with chronic conditions (Stein & Jessop, 1991).

The above studies are models of empirically based interventions that need to be conducted by psychologists and their pediatric colleagues to address such unanswered questions as: What are the critical, most cost-effective elements of comprehensive care for children with various chronic conditions? What are the most effective methods to prevent the psychological morbidity associated with childhood chronic illness? The answers to such questions will be increasingly important in health care reform (see Chapter 16).

7

Research-Related Collaboration

The purpose of this chapter is to describe the special issues that arise in the course of research collaboration with pediatric colleagues. Psychologists and pediatricians can certainly conduct significant research in their respective fields without ever talking to one another. Moreover, collaborative research can have serious drawbacks such as additional time and logistical problems, conflicts of interest and research philosophy among collaborators, and tensions over how to design, analyze, and present research (Drotar, 1989). So why try to collaborate?

ADVANTAGES OF COLLABORATIVE RESEARCH

The necessity for collaborative research is driven by several compelling practical and scientific considerations. The populations of most interest to many pediatric psychologists are pediatricians' patients. In many instances, research cannot be conducted without the pediatricians' permission to contact their patients as well as their active in help in contacting parents of children in their practices to facilitate their participation. Beyond these purely logistic issues, interdisciplinary collaboration is necessary because no single individual or profession can possibly keep abreast of the knowledge and expertise needed to conduct research on complex pediatric conditions, e.g., low-birth-weight infants, chronic illness, etc. Successful conduct of research with pediatric populations requires familiarity with medical aspects of pediatric conditions including pathogenesis, natural history, individual variation in symptoms and severity, as well as special ethical issues (Rae & Fournier, 1986). Because such important areas of knowledge are not emphasized in typical graduate-level research training in psychology, the expertise of pediatricians and other health professionals is often necessary to enhance research design and implementation. Collaborative research also enhances an investigator's ability to secure the financial resources that are necessary to carry out the time-intensive research often needed with pediatric populations. In my experience, grant review committees not only recognize the critical importance of interdisciplinary research with pediatric populations but look with disfavor on research that does not involve a team of collaborators with relevant expertise.

Collaborative research can also produce a level of stimulation, collegial spirit, and mutual sharing that simply cannot be matched in solo research efforts. Moreover, the opportunity to rely on pediatric colleagues allows one to share the considerable burdens involved in designing, funding, and implementing complex research. Beyond the intellectual stimulation and collegial support that can be associated with collaborative research, enhancement of career development is another clear incentive. Research activities can bring positive recognition to psychologists in academic medical school departments. The ability to conduct research independently and to contribute to research identifies the psychologist as someone who can contribute to departmental activities in a variety of ways. In cost-conscious hospital environments, pediatric chairs, hospital administrators, and division leaders also place particular value on funded research. Thus, in academic departments the psychologist (or the pediatrician) who has the capacity to obtain funding for research is a valuable commodity. Although not every psychologist or pediatrician has the ability, interest, or time to develop and manage grant-funded research, many have the capacity and sometimes even the time to develop research in their areas of interest.

Participation in collaborative research has special incentives for pediatricians in academic medical settings who, like their colleagues in pediatric psychology, must contend with strenuous "triple-threat" expectations that they conduct high-volume, high-quality clinical care, teaching, and research. Ledley and Lovejoy's (1993) survey of graduates from a highly respected academic pediatric residency program (Boston Children's Hospital) indicated that the majority of graduates subsequently engaged in a wide range of professional activities, e.g., clinical care, administration, teaching, and research. Most respondents superimposed their research on their clinical activities, engaging in research less than half the time (Ledley & Lovejoy, 1993). Research is even more prohibitive for pediatricians in practice.

Research activities can provide an important if not critical way to offset some of the extraordinary demands of clinical work in pediatric hospital settings. From a personal vantage point, research has been and continues to be of singular importance to my collaborative work, career development, and personal satisfaction. In my setting, collaborative research with pediatricians has also created research training opportunities for undergraduate and graduate students in psychology for more than 20 years (see Chapter 11).

Such important personal benefits notwithstanding, collaborative research may also be critical for the continued development of the scientific knowledge base of the field of pediatric psychology. The rapid growth of this field may be attributed at least in part to the development of clinical methods that have been demonstrated as effective (Roberts, 1992). Clinical research with various pediatric conditions also serves an important heuristic value in identifying clinically important subgroups and developing methods of assessment and intervention approaches (Drotar, 1994). Moreover, there is a continuing need for treatment outcome research, including data concerning the efficacy of collaborative clinical approaches (Roberts, 1992).

MODELS OF RESEARCH-RELATED COLLABORATION

Similar to clinical consultation, research-related collaboration can take many forms depending on the type and level of contact between investigators (Roberts & Wright, 1982). To be most effective, researchers should consider a flexible use of various models that fit with the setting, research question, available populations, and the talents and interests of collaborators (Drotar, 1989). For example, in one typical model of research collaboration, one person assumes primary responsibility for the design and conduct of a research project but uses others' help to consult on issues and help to secure subjects. As an example, some of my recent research in childhood chronic illness has focused on parents' perceptions of family sharing and children's independence concerning treatment-related responsibilities in two chronic illness groups, insulin-dependent diabetes mellitus (IDDM) and cystic fibrosis (CF). To facilitate data collection, I contacted pediatric colleagues in the endocrine and pulmonary divisions for their help in contacting and recruiting families from their patient populations and for suggestions in developing measures of treatment-related responsibilities.

This type of research collaboration works both ways. Psychologists can also lend helpful and much-appreciated expertise in the design and analysis of studies that are largely designed and implemented by pediatric colleagues. One of my colleagues, Terry Stancin, has effectively provided this type of consultation to her medical colleagues on such nonpsychological topics as influences on reinfection following varicella vaccine. Psychologists can also use their expertise in research to teach and inform pediatric faculty and residents about the special design and analytic issues involved in behavioral and developmental pediatric research. For example, interdisciplinary journal club seminars that involve pediatric faculty and residents in reviews of recent research articles can be an effective introduction to research. Most of us feel much more comfortable contributing critiques of someone else's research than we do in having our own work reviewed. For this reason, a journal club can be a safe format in which to introduce concepts and design issues concerning psychological research to pediatric colleagues. A journal club that is organized and led by a psychologist can also serve to advertise one's research interests and expertise to pediatric colleagues.

A more ambitious type of research-related collaboration, which is comparable to the collaborative team model of clinical consultation, involves a high level of mutual responsibility for research design, implementation, data analysis, and writing. This type of collaboration is illustrated by my recent research with Karen Olness, a pediatrician with longstanding interests in psychological development of young children in developing countries (Olness & Torjesen, 1991). For several years, Olness had been involved in research on the natural history of transmission of HIV infection from mother to child in collaboration with physicians at Makerere University in Kampala, the capital city of Uganda, where this condition has reached epidemic proportions (Goodgame, 1990). She recognized the unique potential of research with this population to shed light on the impact of HIV infection on children's psychological development. In contrast to the United States, where HIV infection in young children is confounded with the presence of drug addiction, family instability, and other risk factors, drug addiction is largely nonexistent in Uganda. Moreover, Ugandan infants are born to a stable population of mothers, which not only heightens the feasibility of prospective studies but makes it possible to disentangle the effects of HIV infection on cognitive development from covarying environmental influences. This project began with an invitation from Olness to collaborate on a grant proposal to the National Institutes of Health (NIH). Meeting regularly over a several-month period, we designed a prospective study of the cognitive developmental outcomes of young children (from birth to 24 months) with HIV infection compared to uninfected children, using a comprehensive assessment of cognitive developmental status (e.g., Bayley Scales and Fagan test), neurological status, physical health, and the quality of infants' home environments (Drotar, Fagan, Olness, Hom, Wiznitzer, Marum, Scheurman, & Ndugwa, 1993b). Faculty-level collaboration has also involved Max Wiznitzer, a pediatric neurologist, and Joe Fagan, a developmental psychologist and colleague at Case Western Reserve University. My work on this project has involved two trips to Uganda, which included supervision of Ugandan staff in their administration and scoring of developmental tests and home observations, collaboration with the Ugandan physicians and nursing staff concerning data collection and management, and planning the data analysis. Like other research in the real world, it has had more than its share of frustrating moments. Communications with colleagues in Uganda by phone or FAX are interrupted repeatedly. Coordination of data management has proven to be very difficult. Yet, this collaborative work has been an invaluable learning experience.

FACILITATING RESEARCH-RELATED COLLABORATION

Despite its many advantages, ongoing research-related collaboration with pediatric colleagues is difficult to achieve. Some of the reasons are obvious. Most pediatricians and pediatric psychologists are primarily clinicians who have little time and energy left over to devote to research. The limited time for research may be especially frustrating for psychologists and their pediatric colleagues who have had specialized training and interests in research. In this regard, pediatric psychologists who were surveyed concerning their perceptions of their work environments ranked "not having sufficient time for research" as the top source of work-related dissatisfaction (Drotar *et al.*, 1993a). It may be comforting (in a strange "share the misery" way) for psychologists to know that many pediatricians also feel very frustrated by the difficulties involved in sustaining a research program in academic medical settings (Ledley & Lovejoy, 1993). I know of at least one developmental neurologist who left a full-time faculty position in a department of pediatrics to pursue graduate-level Ph.D. training in developmental psychology primarily because she did not have sufficient time to conduct research in her job.

Other obstacles to collaborative research concern differences in professional style, personality, and attitudes about research (Stein & Jessop, 1988), interests among potential collaborators, and lack of populations in particular settings. Various centers differ considerably in the level of program development and populations in subspecialty areas. Moreover, the strengths of pediatric colleagues in particular settings do not necessarily fit the interests and expertise of psychologists.

Securing Time and Resources

In pediatric settings, lack of sufficient time to conduct research is closely intertwined with the difficulties of obtaining sufficient economic resources to fund data collection and adequately protect investigators' time from the ravages of time-consuming clinical work. Collaborative support from pediatric colleagues may be helpful in obtaining resources to facilitate research in several ways. For example, the availability of a network of pediatric colleagues can extend investigators' access to local and hospital funds and sometimes to staff that can gather data, conduct chart reviews, etc. Enthusiastic collaborators can often manage to accomplish a surprising amount of research by sharing and bootstrapping resources, e.g., time from community volunteers and from students, if they are accessible. Moreover, as pediatric colleagues come to recognize psychologists' expertise in research design and data analysis, they are more likely to invite them to be coinvestigators on their projects, which can also be a way to secure funding and hence time for research. In some instances, pediatric departments can provide small amounts of start-up funds that can be critical to develop projects. Research with pediatric colleagues usually has priority for such funds.

Moreover, collaborators with a strong mutual commitment to a particular area of research can facilitate one another's structuring of time. Colleagues' personal commitments to carve out consistent time for planning and implementing research may make a critical difference in getting a project going or sustaining it. Some colleagues may be more productive by working in tandem because they do not want to let the other person down by failing to complete research-related tasks. In working with colleagues, one can also trade off areas of strength in developing projects; e.g., one person may be better at conceptualization and design, another at data analysis. For this reason, psychologists with strong research interests who are being recruited for positions in medical settings should consider whether a prospective job setting has populations, opportunities for local funding, and interested, willing, and talented pediatric collaborators in their chosen area of research.

Developing Support for Collaborative Research

Psychologists may also find that their progress in developing collaborative research with pediatric colleagues may depend at least in part on the quality of their support from their psychologist. If they are available and interested, senior mentors who are successful researchers can provide support by introducing a junior person to the world of grant proposals, giving tips on time management, and providing advice on research design.

Psychologists who are interested in developing research careers also need to secure strong support from their division heads and administrators. The heads of the pediatric psychology programs reviewed in Chapter 8 have managed to use various strategies to obtain a range of support for research in their divisions, e.g., research assistant time, reduced clinical load. In my own career, the strong support of Charlie Malone, who was chief of Child Psychiatry for a number of years at Case Western Reserve University, was influential by strongly advocating that I secure time for research and focus on a specific population and by helping to develop funding for a series of projects that laid the groundwork for my research concerning FTT (Drotar, 1988). In most medical settings, one has to advocate clearly and consistently for one's research to pediatric colleagues and hospital administrators. Prospects for future research grant funding can provide considerable incentive for pediatric chairs and division heads to support faculty research efforts.

In my experience, more formal strategies may also facilitate the development of collaborative research. For example, small working groups of potential collaborators who meet regularly to discuss research projects in an area of mutual interest may be very helpful. Such groups can be free ranging, e.g., focusing on presentation of research ideas and work in progress. However, structured groups that are focused on a particular task are maximally efficient. Writers' workshops, seminars, and retreats can also be an effective method of stimulating productivity among researchers. Hekelman, Gilchrist, Glover, Olness, and Zyzanski (in press) described a model for enhancing research productivity that included a seminar in which physicians faculty were given didactic training on writing and publication and prepared an outline of a paper. This was followed 8 weeks later by an all-day workshop on manuscript critique and practice in writing with feedback from senior research advisors. Participation in this series facilitated the publication of peer-reviewed papers by 11 of 45 participants. Karen Olness (personal communication, Jan. 10, 1994) has utilized a retreat format to help faculty participants develop a specific writing project, e.g., proposal, draft of a manuscript. Participants distribute drafts of their writing for critique by workshop participants. Writers then produce additional drafts followed by multiple critiques. The combination of social support and critique in such a group format can be a very powerful method of facilitating the development of writing skills and completion of manuscripts.

Starting Small and Ending Up Big

Research collaborations in pediatric settings generally do not spring up overnight but reflect the mutual persistence of interested colleagues who gradually build on their work in a step-by-step manner. In some cases, successful research-related collaborations develop from a series of mutually satisfying experiences in other activities, especially clinical consultation. For example, my research concerning children with cystic fibrosis (CF) and their families developed from several years of clinical consultation with physicians in the pediatric pulmonary department at

Rainbow Babies' & Children's Hospital. Shortly after I arrived in this setting, members of this group asked me to evaluate and provide intervention for a wide range of problems that were identified in children and adolescents with CF, e.g., difficulties with adherence, learning problems, problems with depression. Such clinical experiences led us to wonder whether the nature and severity of psychological difficulties encountered among patients who were referred for psychological consultation were generalizable across the broader population of children and adolescents with CF who were followed at this center. With funding from the Cleveland chapter of the CF foundation that was facilitated by one of my colleagues (Carl Doershuk), we implemented a controlled study of the psychological adjustment of children and adolescents as rated by parents and teachers (Drotar *et al.*, 1982). Eventually, this collaboration supported several student dissertation research projects, including a home observational study of the relationship of family functioning to psychological adjustment in children with CF (Kucia, Drotar, Doershuk, Stern, Boat, & Matthews, 1979), a study of the correlates of coping and adjustment in young adults with CF (Moise, Drotar, Doershuk, & Stern, 1987), and studies of the impact of home apnea monitoring on family adaptation (Phipps & Drotar, 1990). My collaboration with this physician group has continued right up until the present in studies of parenting practices (Ievers, Drotar, Dahms, Doershuk & Stern, 1994) and family sharing of treatment-related responsibilities in chronic illness populations (Drotar & Ievers, 1994).

Cooperative research with pediatric subspecialty groups can be particularly efficient for several reasons (Drotar, 1989). Many pediatric subspecialists prefer to collaborate with "their own" psychologist who is not only interested in their patients but has special expertise with these populations. In some cases, the support staff associated with many subspecialty research and clinical care programs can facilitate programmatic research that addresses a series of questions. It is no accident that some productive research programs in pediatric psychology have focused on specialized populations. Suzanne Bennett-Johnson's research on juvenile diabetes at the University of Florida is one primary example (Johnson, Silverstein, Rosenbloom, Carter, & Cunningham, 1986).

PROBLEMATIC ISSUES IN RESEARCH-RELATED COLLABORATION

Similar to interdisciplinary practice, research-related collaboration is not always a smooth or mutually satisfying process. In my experience, serious collaborative strain can be created by ambiguities and/or differences in role expectations and by struggles for control and ownership of the research. Although the lines of authority and responsibility for some projects can be clearly demarcated, e.g., when one investigator is consulting to another, they are not so clear in projects in which collaborators have strong, vested interests and where ideas, resources, and responsibilities are freely shared. In such circumstances, disagreements concerning the design and conduct of research, authorship credit, and publication outlet can be particularly problematic (Drotar, 1989).

The interdependence of research collaboration can also prove frustrating. Progress depends on collaborators' abilities and willingness to fulfill their fair share of the many responsibilities involved in developing and implementing a research project, e.g., talking to patients about participating in the project, writing a description of the proposed study for research review committees, supplying relevant clinical information, interviewing families, working with data, writing the findings up for presentation and publication. The momentum of research studies can be severely hampered by long delays in completing shared tasks. Moreover, collaborators have different standards and expectations for the quality and promptness of task completion as well as differences in work styles (Stein & Jessop, 1988). Researchers who feel they have put in much more time and effort than their colleagues may become very frustrated with their colleagues. Although it is difficult to discuss mutual expectations and frustrations about performance in research with colleagues, such dialogue may be necessary if collaboration is to be successful.

Other collaborative conflicts relate to discrepancies in professional training and philosophy that create different expectations about research design, methods, and credit for scientific contributions (Stein & Jessop, 1988). For example, some physicians are frustrated by the lack of a "gold standard" to measure psychological outcomes (Drotar, 1989) and may prefer clinical ratings of adjustment or interviews that have apparent clinical relevance and validity. Others may show unwarranted trust that psychological tests provide an unbiased or "true" measure of a child's or parent's feelings about their illness, family situation, etc. On the other hand, psychologists may be surprised by problems with medical diagnostic procedures or inconsistent data concerning the efficacy of some medical treatments.

The following example illustrates such collaborative tensions. Based on his clinical experience, a pediatric endocrinologist was convinced that children with hypopituitarism had a "deviant" body image. He felt that objective psychological measures would be less sensitive than interviews to assess children's attitudes toward their bodies. However, the psychologist felt that data from an unstandardized clinical interview would not contribute valid information. After several heated discussions, the investigators agreed to include data from psychological tests *and* clinical interviews in their proposed study. Their final decision to assess the reliability of the clinical interview *and* its correspondence with psychological test data provided information that was useful to both of them (Drotar, 1989).

Collaborative research can also generate heated conflicts about the most appropriate way to disseminate findings, e.g., choice of professional meetings, publication outlet, and authorship. Researchers who prefer to publish their findings in a journal that results in recognition and credit from their professional peers may regard publication in another profession's journal as less than desirable. Not surprisingly, pediatricians prefer publishing in major pediatric journals, e.g., *Pediatrics*, and presenting findings at *their* meetings, e.g., Society for Pediatric Research, whereas psychologists prefer to publish in outlets such as the *Journal of Pediatric Psychology* and present their work to psychologists' meetings. There is no easy way for collaborators to make decisions concerning outlets for publication or presentation of research findings. However, among trusted colleagues, effective compromise may be achieved by selecting a professionally neutral interdisciplinary publication, alternating publications in different professional journals, deciding on the "best" outlet for publication of their paper on the basis of research content or journal circulation, or "splitting" the data to be presented and/or published to psychologist and pediatric audiences. However, at all costs, collaborators should avoid the unethical resolution of this problem by submitting essentially the same data set to two different publication outlets (APA, 1992).

Decisions concerning authorship credit, e.g., whether work contributed to a research project warrants credit for authorship versus an acknowledgement, and the order of authors can also be a source of collegial conflict. Irrespective of professional guidelines (e.g., APA, 1992; International Committee of Medical Journal Editors, 1985), some collaborators may apply strongly held but idiosyncratic expectations concerning receipt of credit for their contributions to a research project. Given the potential for conflict involving decisions concerning authorship credit, collaborators should decide on authorship early in the development of their projects, rather than leave this decision until it is time to publish the findings (Burman, 1982).

FUTURE DIRECTIONS

Training for Collaborative Research

Collaborative research with pediatricians presents special practical problems and requires a specialized knowledge base that outstrips the standard fare of traditional graduate training programs in psychology. To equip students to manage such problems, specialized training experiences will be necessary. These include (among others) didactic teaching concerning strategies and problems in developing research-related collaborations with pediatricians, close involvement of pediatricians in mentorship, and experience in research with pediatricians (Drotar, 1989) (see Chapter 11).

Using Research to Develop New Clinical Programs

One very interesting and important function of collaborative research in pediatric settings is to provide data that can facilitate the development and adoption of intervention programs for pediatric populations. Maureen Black's experiences in helping to develop the Growth and Nutrition Clinic (GNC) in the Department of Pediatrics at the University of Maryland provides an instructive example (M. Black, personal communication, Dec. 1, 1993).

The GNC was initially established to evaluate and treat children with failure to thrive (FTT) as part of a grant from the Bureau of Maternal and Child Health to evaluate the effects of home intervention on the growth and development of infants and young children under the age of 2 years with nonorganic FTT. This project provided comprehensive assessment (pediatric, social work, nutritional, and developmental) and follow-up of all children enrolled in the program and their families. All families received at least two home visits, and half the families received home intervention designed to promote adaptive parenting and parent–child interaction. An objective evaluation indicated significant improvements in the children's weight for age and weight for height over an 18-month period in both intervention groups. These data, which were based on a sample of 145 children enrolled during a 3-year period, suggested that this multidisciplinary, family-oriented approach of the GNC was an effective strategy to manage the problems of growth and nutrition in this population (Black, Dubowitz, Hutcheson, Berenson-Howard, & Starr, 1994). These findings were presented to the Maryland Department of Health and Mental Hygiene (DHMH) along with a proposal to provide evaluation and treatment to children from birth through age 3 with poor growth, irrespective of etiology. Convinced by these findings, the DHMH staff authorized an agreement for funding through purchase of a care program as part of an expanded Episodic, Periodic Screening Diagnosis and Treatment Program (EPSDT). Additional funding from the state was necessary because the clinic could not be maintained through hospital resources. The majority of families who were enrolled in the GNC either received Medicaid or were uninsured. The funds provided by the state DHMH program provided sufficient resources for the GNC staff to evaluate 50 new families per year and to provide ongoing treatment. Services are now provided by a collaborative team that includes psychology, pediatric gastroenterology, nutrition, social work, and nursing. Each child receives an average of eight follow-up visits. The clinic has developed collaboration with community agencies. Comprehensive clinical data collected on children's growth, family demographics, developmental status, and family interaction during feeding provide information that is used in clinical management.

Black and her colleagues' experiences in developing comprehensive services for a difficult-to-reach population based on collaborative research provide one model for the integration of collaborative research and practice in an academic medical setting. Schroeder, Christophersen, and their colleagues' research (see Chapter 4) provide other models for integrating psychological research with pediatric practice.

Using Research to Develop Pediatric Psychology Programs

Productive collaborative research programs can also facilitate the development of pediatric psychology programs in academic medical settings (see Chapter 8). In some instances, descriptive research on services, consumer satisfaction, and outcomes can help to convince recalcitrant hospital administrators of the need to develop or expand pediatric psychology services. In all of this work, an important and continuing goal is to convince pediatric colleagues and administrators that psychological research is an excellent investment that can reap dividends in improved patient care, more satisfied faculty, and enhanced local and national visibility of programs. Moreover, research concerning the efficacy of psychological services will undoubtedly assume increasing importance as a function of managed care (see Chapters 10 and 16).

8

Developing Pediatric Psychology Programs in Academic Medical Settings

Programmatic collaboration can be defined as cooperative work (services, research, or teaching) among psychologists and pediatricians that occurs over an extended period of time for the purpose of maintaining, expanding, or improving teaching, research, or service programs. This type of collaboration may occur among individual colleagues or among larger groups, e.g., between a division of psychology and a pediatric subspecialty. The features of continuity, purpose, and planning distinguish programmatic collaboration from the day-to-day cooperative work that occurs among colleagues. Programmatic collaboration may be highly focused, e.g., developing a service with a pediatric subspecialty group, or more comprehensive, e.g., planning activities of psychologists in a department of pediatrics.

There are relatively few descriptions of programmatic collaboration between pediatricians and psychologists, especially in academic medical settings. Schroeder and Mann (1991) have described such collaboration in a community practice setting. To address this need, this chapter describes issues concerning programmatic collaboration, examples of pediatric psychology programs in different settings, and implications.

OBSTACLES TO PROGRAMMATIC COLLABORATION

Problematic Communication

Program development and management require a level of administrative and communicative skill that is very difficult to achieve, especially within the organizational, time, and economic constraints of many medical settings. Consider a mythical collaborative scenario that illustrates communication problems among administrators and their staff. A pediatric oncologist is interested in expanding her bone marrow transplantation program. She wants the psychology staff to provide psychosocial support for children in the program and strongly communicates this expectation to the chief psychologist. Not wanting to offend his pediatric colleague, the chief psychologist assigns one of his staff to the oncology service. However, the psychologist who drew this assignment is not at all thrilled with the extra work. This ambivalence contributes to a low volume of service, which eventually generates complaints from the staff. The chief of oncology becomes very frustrated and bypasses the chief psychologist to complain to the chair of pediatrics about the "problems" in psychology. Already unsure about how the psychologists contribute to departmental programs, the chair decides to terminate the psychologist's involvement and approach social work about covering the service. Not surprisingly, the psychology staff are up in arms.

Problems in Administrative Organization

Problematic interdisciplinary communication at a program level can be intensified by complex administrative arrangements such as appointments in multiple departments and allegiances to multiple organizations, e.g., hospital versus medical school. Such organizational problems can also contribute to diffusion of responsibility, confusion, and staff conflict. One fairly typical administrative arrangement is for the psychologists who work in a department of pediatrics to have their major administrative appointments in a department of psychiatry. As the first psychologist hired to work full time in a pediatric teaching hospital, my major academic and hospital administrative appointment was in the department of psychiatry. I soon learned that responsibilities for securing such niceties as office space, furniture, and secretarial support had not been worked out between the departments. Given some ingenuity, initiative, and most especially the ability to scavenge, I eventually found temporary space with the help of pediatric colleagues. Soon we moved into a new building where psychology office space had been arranged but furniture had not. Fortunately, I was able to tag some leftover furniture to use in the interim. The next hurdle was secretarial support. Some support for typing reports and billing was available in psychiatry. However, this was not only inconvenient but was inadequate to meet the needs of an expanding psychology service. During one of many conversations with the pediatric hospital administrator about these problems, I was informed that I was in the "gray area" between the two departments (pediatrics and psychiatry). Although this was true, somehow it was not especially comforting.

In some settings, divided administrative authority for psychology between pediatrics and psychiatry can confuse and disrupt decision making. Leaders of departments of pediatrics are understandably invested in having authority and control over individuals and programs in *their* department and may become frustrated when this is not possible. Moreover, splitting administrative authority between departments of pediatrics and psychiatry may create a situation in which the heads of each of these departments negotiate with one another rather than directly with the psychologists, a situation that not only disrupts effective planning but undermines professional autonomy.

In some situations, the fate of psychologists in pediatrics may be determined by events and resource problems in other departments that have little to do with the quality or quantity of work with their pediatric colleagues. For example, consider the following mythical worst-case scenario. A new chair of psychiatry is hired whose main research and clinical agenda involves biological psychiatry. In the midst of a budget crunch, the new chair unilaterally decides to reduce the staff of psychologists in pediatrics without regard for their history of collaboration and program development, thus causing considerable outrage among psychologists and their pediatric colleagues.

It is, of course, possible to administer a pediatric psychology program in a department of psychiatry. However, to make this arrangement work, extraordinary efforts and individuals are required.

Lack of Resources

Modern pediatric hospitals must struggle to make ends meet in a climate of complex and shifting patterns of reimbursability rates, responsibilities to provide care for indigent patients at an economic loss, shrinking birth rates and "markets," and competition from local hospitals (Dana & May, 1986). Needing to support the salaries of faculty and house staff, academic teaching institutions face extraordinary economic problems and difficult if not impossible dilemmas in balancing human need versus cost efficacy in developing new programs and/or expanding existing services (Halpern, 1988). Profitability often shapes departmental priorities for expansion. When psychology programs are viewed under the hard lens of economic costs versus benefits, it is easy to see why they are very difficult to fund and develop and why successful administrators of these programs must have (or develop) a strong entrepreneurial bent and many allies among their pediatric colleagues. Psychologists at many university-based teaching hospitals see large numbers of indigent patients but typically do not admit patients to hospitals. Pediatric psychologists also provide important but nonreimbursable services such as phone contact with parents and teachers, school visits and consultation, discussions of treatment planning, and follow-up with pediatricians. Psychological services are not usually reimbursed by insurance companies at 100%, if they are reimbursed at all.

Conflicts among Psychologists

Despite considerable external constraints, some of the greatest impediments to program development in pediatric settings can come from within. Psychologists in pediatric settings may have very different opinions about strategies and priority areas for program development. Conflict and divisiveness among psychologists may also be intensified by the subspecialized emphasis of pediatric settings, diverse interests, competition for tenure, scarce resources, and/or lack of leadership or effective authority. If psychologists try to improve their individual positions without considering the impact on their colleagues, program development and morale may eventually suffer. Moreover, infighting among psychologists consumes considerable emotional energy that could otherwise be devoted to productive program planning.

INGREDIENTS OF SUCCESSFUL PROGRAMMATIC COLLABORATION

In the "ideal" professional setting, pediatricians and psychologists develop their clinical care, teaching, and research programs through a shared vision and conjoint planning. The features of such persistent, cooperative planning are illustrated by an alternative scenario for psychologist–pediatrician collaboration, again taken from a mythical, idealized hospital setting. In this case, the chief psychologist did not make a unilateral decision concerning the oncologist's request for increased psychological services but discussed the request with his staff. After some discussion, it was decided that one of the psychologists would be able to free up some time by reducing some general service responsibilities. However, the group was very concerned that even this expanded time commitment would not adequately cover the needs of children and families. The chief psychologist informed the oncologist of these concerns and inquired about funding to support the position. The oncologist discussed the financial plight of her division and the mounting pressures on her staff for increased service. Her bottom line answer was a polite but clear "no way." However, because both parties were convinced of the importance of this new position, the issue did not end there. They agreed to approach the department chair, the hospital administrator, and a local foundation to discuss the need and funding prospects for this position. Following extended discussions and more complete documentation of the need for this service, an additional 30% of a salary was freed up for a time-limited period, which, together with the anticipated reallocation of staff time, now amounted to a half-time position. The chief psychologist and oncologist agreed that this was still not adequate. However, given the compelling need for the service, they decided to proceed. They also agreed to gather detailed data concerning services, reimbursement patterns, and staff and family satisfaction and to explore alternative funding sources.

It is instructive to review the interprofessional transactions in this vignette. First, the oncologist did not make a unilateral assumption that services would be provided but discussed the problem with the chief psychologist, who in turn discussed the implications with his staff. Although neither had sufficient resources for the position, these collaborators worked together to develop resources for the position they wanted. This vignette illustrates several ingredients of successful programmatic collaboration, including pediatricians' recognition of psychologists' potential contributions to hospital programs, administrative clarity and support, financial resources, and leadership.

Departmental Recognition of Psychologists' Contributions

To make programmatic collaboration effective, colleagues need to recognize and appreciate one another's professional contributions (see Chapter 2). Many of the heads of pediatric departments have spent their professional lives in research and in specialties such as infectious disease or neonatology, where psychologists' contributions are hardly a household word. Moreover, administrators of large pediatric departments and hospitals have many needs to fill and crises to solve. Consequently, the burden is on psychologists to familiarize their pediatric colleagues with their work and to encourage them to advocate the need for psychological service, teaching, or research programs with hospital and departmental administrators.

Psychology programs generally achieve recognition and visibility through responsive clinical consultation and a broad range of teaching and research contributions. Because of their small numbers relative to pediatric colleagues, pediatric psychologists generally need to work very hard and make judicious choices about where to invest their limited staff resources. Hence, priorities should be given to programs that have enthusiastic pediatric supporters and show potential for future development.

Administrators of psychology programs also need to ensure that their department chair, relevant division heads, and hospital administrators are clearly and continually informed about their staff's contributions. For this reason, written reports and face-to-face meetings are not merely informative but are critical to teach pediatric administrators about the range of psychologists' contributions, highlight successful programs or individuals, and identify new teaching, service, or research needs that justify program expansion.

Clarity of Administrative Communication and Decision Making

Effective programmatic collaboration requires clear and direct communication among the administrative leaders in pediatrics and psychology as well as between these leaders and the staff who are working in the "trenches." Unless psychologists participate in decisions concerning program development and deployment of their activities, it may be very difficult for them to sustain the high level of professional initiative that is necessary to sustain successful program development. At the same time, psychologists' activities also need to be closely integrated with and accountable to departmental and/or hospital goals and programs. Close and open communication among pediatric psychologists and pediatricians at all levels is necessary to achieve and sustain the difficult balance between professional autonomy and accountability.

Leadership and Power

Effective leadership from psychologists and pediatricians is another critical ingredient in the difficult recipe for effective programmatic collaboration. Leaders of pediatric psychology programs need to have a high level of energy, ingenuity to develop and organize new programs, and the ability to provide support and guidance to their colleagues. This is clearly a tall order to fill. Beyond these personal virtues and talents, the administrative leader of a psychology program must be acknowledged as such by other administrators and pediatric colleagues. Otherwise, he or she will have little negotiating power. Chairpersons of medical school departments generally wield a great deal of influence. Consequently, their support and advocacy are critical for the continued development of all programs within their purview, including psychology.

Teamwork and Group Support

Although support from pediatric colleagues is clearly important to successful program development, support from one's own colleagues may be just as critical, if not more so. Similar to their pediatric colleagues, many psychologists in academic settings are called upon to develop teaching, service, and research programs (the legendary triple threat). Legends notwithstanding, all but the most talented and/or driven of psychologists will usually not be able to achieve consistent excellence in all of these areas. On the other hand, if they work as a team, a group of psychologists may be able to achieve a successful balance of teaching, research, and clinical activities within their departmental programs. All but the most goal-directed and independent of psychologists may require some support from their colleagues to manage the high level of work-related demands in medical settings. Colleagues can provide an important source of professional identity as well as collaborators in teaching, services, or research programs.

Developing Economic Resources

The level of economic resources that can be made available to develop and sustain a pediatric psychology program is in many ways the most critical ingredient of programmatic collaboration. No single revenue source will ensure continuation or expansion of a pediatric psychology program. Consequently, psychologists in pediatric settings need to combine their professional strengths to generate diverse sources of income from clinical care, teaching, and research and to marshal support from pediatric departments, hospital, and, where possible, state and local funds to sustain their work.

Examples of Program Development in Academic Medical Settings

Substantial local variations in hospitals, administrative structures, and influential figures (e.g., chairs of departments) limit generalizations about factors that characterize successful program development in pediatric psychology. Pediatric psychologists will sometimes swap collaborative war stories and fiascoes at professional meetings. However, it is more difficult to obtain information about program content and development. In order to obtain information, I used the informal, admittedly biased strategy of writing to heads and/or influential figures in psychology programs in academic medical settings who I knew had somehow managed to expand their programs. I asked them to describe their programs and to contribute some thoughts about what enhanced program development in their settings. I focused on divisions of pediatric psychology in academic medical settings because these programs employ significant numbers of psychologists (Drotar *et al.*, 1993a). Here is a brief description of four such programs, followed by a discussion of implications.

Department of Pediatrics, University of Iowa College of Medicine, Dennis Harper, Professor. The Division of Pediatric Psychology is located in the Department of Pediatrics at the University of Iowa Hospitals and Clinics and consists of six full-time psychologists with faculty appointments, two staff psychologists, four graduate assistants, and two predoctoral and one postdoctoral trainee (D. Harper, personal communication, Dec. 30, 1993). An associated group of five and one-half staff psychologists at the University Hospital School, Division of Developmental Disabilities, brings the number of psychologists in this setting to 14. This program features specialized services rather than general consultation. Specialized clinics are offered in neuropsychological consultation, learning disability, attention deficit hyperactivity disorder, acute and chronic health impairments, psychosomatic complaints and pain management, behavior management, oncology, adolescent adjustment concerns, and a feeding/eating disorder consultation service. Various specialized services are also provided as part of a multidisciplinary team at the University Hospital School for children and young adults with developmental disorders, etc.

This program evolved from a long history of collaboration, now spanning nearly 30 years. This is one of the longest-running programs in pediatric psychology, and a brief account of its evolution is instructive. In 1965, two pediatricians, one the departmental chair and the other a director of a statewide community-based health care program for children, encouraged Vinton Rowley, then a faculty psychologist in child psychiatry at the University of Iowa, to develop a pediatric psychology service program within the Department of Pediatrics. Academic appointments for psychologists originated and have been maintained in the Department of Pediatrics ever since.

From 1965 to now, this program has strongly emphasized service. One important feature has been the consultation provided by psychologists in communities throughout the state of Iowa. Additional staff psychologists were added in 1965–1971. By 1980, there were seven faculty members, all based on "hard money" from the Department of Pediatrics. Over time, this program's clinical care has become increasingly specialized, focusing on particular disabilities and/or health-related problems. Research productivity and grant-funded research have become increasingly important, not only to departmental activities but to faculty development and tenure. All psychology faculty have some external grant support and are expected to maintain such funding. In some cases, research protocols have been designed to fit into existing clinical services to maximize efficiency of time and effort and thereby have increased research productivity.

This faculty has also had a long-standing, strong commitment to graduate medical and psychology education and assumes responsibility for its own training programs within the medical school and for psychology graduate students. Teaching of medical students has occurred at all levels (first-year students through residents to fellows), and multiple teaching (didactic and clinical) opportunities are offered for many years. Graduate students in psychology have been incorporated into the clinical service programs to enhance their capacity to provide teaching and supervision. Several faculty have appointments in other graduate departments. All faculty regularly cochair dissertations and participate in master's/doctoral committees in multiple departments throughout the graduate departments of the University of Iowa.

In looking toward the future of this program, Harper noted the need for increasing diversity of fiscal support for psychologists not only from the Department of Pediatrics but from service and research. To help meet their research objectives, several faculty members have successfully developed clinical research as part of their daily efforts. A current trend is to employ additional staff psychologists to assist with clinical service throughout the hospital.

Department of Pediatrics, University of Arkansas for Medical Sciences, Nicholas Long, Associate Professor and Director. Pediatric psychology in the Department of Pediatrics at Arkansas Children's Hospital and the University of Arkansas for Medical Sciences is an example of a newer pediatric psychology program that has achieved rapid programmatic growth and a fivefold increase in psychologists over a 5-year period (1987–1992) (N. Long, personal communication, Nov. 4, 1993). This faculty includes 15 full-time Ph.D.-level members in tenure-track positions. Five masters'-level psychological examiners, who provide psychoeducational and developmental testing, complement the services of this group. The staff also includes a full-time research assistant funded by the Department of Pediatrics. All psychologists have their administrative appointments in this department at the University of Arkansas for Medical Sciences. Pediatric psychology was originally part of a section of developmental pediatrics but has been a separate section since 1989.

Eight psychologists are in a general section of pediatric psychology that is on an equal administrative footing with other sections of the department. The other seven are housed physically and administratively in separate sections of the department: adolescent medicine, behavioral pediatrics, and child abuse. However, the director of pediatric psychology also serves as director of psychological services and hires and is engaged in faculty development for all psychologists. Long described this structural organization as a compromise between maintaining a solid core identity of pediatric psychology and addressing the need to tailor services, teaching, and research to individual pediatric subspecialty programs.

The development of this program has been facilitated by a diverse package of fiscal support to the Department of Pediatrics, including psychology, that includes state-supported health and human services programs (e.g., state Department of Human Services contracts, enhanced Medicaid reimbursements, and Title XX. Consultants hired by the Department of Pediatrics assist all sections including the pediatric psychology group in identifying and maximizing funding sources for proposed and ongoing programs. However, even with such support, the Psychology Department relies to a large extent on clinical revenues to sustain itself and develop new programs. The program's productivity has been enhanced by the use of full-time master's-level clinicians (psychology examiners) who provide testing. With the clinical revenues they generate, these examiners cover their salary as well as a portion of the faculty member's salary under whom they bill. This arrangement gives the faculty psychologists more time to devote to academic work.

The psychology staff work very closely with pediatric subspecialties, e.g., neonatology, hematology, adolescent medicine, and developmental pediatrics. The psychology faculty's diverse tenure-track appointments, e.g., clinical scientist, clinical educator, allow some to specialize more in clinical than research activities. Irrespective of their tenure track, most faculty members have active research programs. This group has also been very active in pediatric residency training and in providing continuing education for professionals, presentations for parents, and community media exposure, as well as in committee work within the hospital. It has been more difficult to involve graduate students in psychology. Although there is no doctoral-level psychology program in the area, postdoctoral training is offered in general pediatric psychology and neuropsychology.

Faculty productivity has been enhanced by a research assistant provided by the Department of Pediatrics, who collects and codes data. This has allowed faculty members to collect pilot data and hence be more successful in obtaining extramural research funding. Long anticipates that future expansion of pediatric psychology in his setting may not be as dramatic as it has been over the past 6 years but that this program will continue to be viable.

Children's Hospital of Columbus and Ohio State University, Tom Linscheid, Professor and Director. Pediatric psychology at Children's Hospital of Columbus has also experienced active growth over the past 10 years. Tom Linscheid (personal communication, Jan. 7, 1994) noted that eight full-time Ph.D.-level staff members of his psychology department have diverse activities and appointments. Five of these positions are Ohio State University (OSU) employees with full tenure status in pediatrics. Three also have joint appointments with the Department of Psychology at OSU. Such joint appointments have provided access to graduate students for assistance in research and revenue-generating clinical activities. The remaining three Ph.D.-level psychologists have "clinical line" positions in which they are employees of Children's Hospital and have a clinical (nontenure, noncompensatory) appointment in the Department of Pediatrics at OSU. These clinical positions involve a higher clinical load, with teaching and especially research less emphasized. These diverse appointments reflect the very different activities of these psychologists and promote flexibility of their contributions to the overall program. The entire pediatric psychology staff, including secretaries, psychometrician, postdoctoral fellows, interns, faculty, and research assistants (three of whom are supported full-time by grants), numbers 21.5 full-time positions.

Despite diversity in their activities and appointments, all psychologists are administered in the Department of Psychology that is funded by the Children's Hospital. This arrangement contrasts with that of the two previous programs. Based on an agreement established with the chair of pediatrics, financial support, operating expense, travel, supplies, etc. come from the Children's Hospital budget process. This Department of Psychology is also a division within the OSU Department of Pediatrics. To foster their professional allegiance and identity, all psychologists are clearly identified with the psychology department. However, those with specialty expertise may be assigned to pediatric divisions, e.g., hematology/ oncology, endocrine, for their primary clinical and research activities.

Psychologists in this program have been heavily involved in psychological training activities. The group has an APA-approved internship in pediatric psychology, which is one of few such programs in the country. The internship program also includes a specialty in clinical child/community mental health that is shared jointly with Children's Hospital Guidance Centers and has a total of six interns. This program also supports four postdoctoral fellows, two in neuropsychology, one in pediatric psychology/ child abuse, and one in pediatric psychology/developmental disabilities. Postdoctoral training positions are supported through either service contracts, salary savings based on faculty release time from grants, or fee for service.

This program also has several active specialized clinical and research programs in neuropsychology, sexual abuse, etc. Faculty in this program are active researchers, and some have external research funding. A clinical service program for children and families who are victims of sexual abuse is expanding to treat adolescent offenders and sexually acting-out children. Primarily staffed by master's-level psychologists and social workers, this is strictly a fee-for-services program.

Alfred I. DuPont Institute, Wayne Adams, Associate Professor and Director. Pediatric psychology at The Alfred I. DuPont Institute Children's Hospital of the Nemours Foundation, Wilmington, Delaware, has flourished in a somewhat different setting, a private, nonprofit 100-bed teaching hospital. This psychology division underwent a significant expansion from 1976, when there were only two full-time psychologists who provided developmental evaluations as part of a multidisciplinary child diagnostic clinic, to the current roster of 10 full-time psychologists, one psychology assistant, three interns, and one learning disabilities specialist.

In this setting, the Division of Psychology is on equal administrative footing with other divisions within the Department of Pediatrics. This arrangement is a recent change from an initial structure in which psychology was considered a hospital department (such as social work or occupational therapy) as opposed to a medical department. This program features a flexible administrative arrangement that is both centralized and closely tied to individual specialties, especially GI, endocrinology, rheumatology, neurology, nephrology, developmental medicine, and neonatal intensive care. This arrangement has facilitated collaborative clinical program development and research efforts. Although most of the 10 psychologists have their central responsibilities in the psychology division and have adjoining offices, three work full-time and are administratively, physically, and fiscally associated with the hospital's 40-bed Division of Rehabilitation. Some psychologists are in positions of leadership. For example, a psychologist heads the hospital's clinic for children with attention deficit disorder. Others colead an obesity clinic and head injury program.

The main emphasis of this program is clinical service, especially outpatient services, including assessment and psychotherapy. The division is of sufficient size that individual staff can emphasize clinical service, teaching, or research. Psychologists are involved in each of these areas, but clinical care predominates. Teaching includes supervision of psychology interns and a new training module for pediatric residents. The hospital is affiliated with Jefferson Medical College, and some staff have academic appointments. Research is encouraged by an internally funded small-grants program. One externally funded training grant supports the psychology internship program. The hospital's research department currently funds a research assistant who is primarily assigned to division staff.

Programmatic expansion has been slow but steady and has been largely facilitated by providing services that have been responsive to pediatric referrals. According to Adams (W. Adams, personal communication, May 25, 1993), collaborating physicians have been advocates for the growth and parity of the psychology division. Moreover, patient satisfaction has also played an important role in the growth of the program.

COMMON THEMES IN PROGRAM DEVELOPMENT

Psychologists in each of these programs have struggled with such difficult questions as the following: What is the best way to marshal support with colleagues for expansion? How does one convince a hospital administration to support expansion? How can these programs be funded? How can one preserve critical elements of existing programs while developing new ones? All of these programs have managed to develop and expand in a difficult economic climate. Despite the diversity of settings and programs, some generalizations can be made. Each of these have developed high-volume, high-quality clinical services that have been highly visible and responsive to the needs of pediatric faculty. Each of these contributors also noted that the support of the departmental chair and pediatric faculty was critical to the development of their programs. Finally, each of these programs appears to have the following characteristics: diversity of funding sources and activities, a strong administrative identity as psychologists, and continuity of energetic, supportive leadership.

Diversity of Funding Sources and Activities

Diversity has always been a strength of pediatric psychology as a professional discipline, and these pediatric psychology programs are no exception. Each of the programs has combined a strong emphasis on clinical services with teaching, research, and, in some instances, community service programs. In order to continue their diverse agendas, these programs have developed multiple funding sources and have added additional staff, e.g., research assistants or master's-level psychologists, to support their work. In accord with their interests and activities, psychologists in each of these programs have diverse appointments and activities and flexible allocation of clinical, research, and teaching activities.

Core Administrative Identity as Psychologists

Although the above programs have different administrative arrangements, all have a core administrative identity as a psychology staff. In each of these programs, the director of psychology plays a primary role in decisions concerning the hiring, deployment, and administration of psychologists. These programs have responded to the needs of pediatric faculty for specialized research and clinical programs without giving up administrative control of pediatric subspecialists. Finally, each of these programs is clearly identified with and administered in a department of pediatrics. Although psychologists in these programs maintain relationships with colleagues in departments of psychiatry, administration of these programs is separate and independent from psychiatry.

Energetic, Supportive Leadership

Although these pediatric psychologists did not emphasize their roles in program development, my reading suggested that the growth of their programs was related in no small measure to their efforts. Each of them has provided leadership to enhance the professional development of the staff in their settings, helped to develop new programs, and worked with departmental administrators to secure and maintain funding for psychological activities. All have been mindful of the need to develop programs that not only meet the needs of pediatricians, children, and families but strongly support the profession of psychology.

FUTURE DIRECTIONS

Programmatic collaboration and consultation and administration are highly important but largely invisible activities of pediatric psychologists. Consequently, one of the important future tasks is to make these critical, behind-the-scenes activities more visible. The four pediatric psychology programs that are described here are certainly not the only models. Other programs have developed and sustained innovative service, teaching, and research programs. It will be important to describe pediatric psychology programs systematically in a range of settings along such dimensions as longevity, staffing activities, volume of clinical services, sources and amounts of salary, research funding, administrative organization, etc. Such information would be of special utility to the directors of pediatric psychology programs who want to compare their programs with others and to administrators who want to develop or expand programs in their settings. This chapter has suggested some hypotheses about effective programmatic strategies. However, additional "case studies" of programs across a range of settings are clearly needed.

Although many pediatric psychologists report that they are involved in some type of administration (Drotar *et al.*, 1993a), very few, if any, receive formal training in these activities. Consequently, important administrative tasks must be learned "on the job" and often by trial and error. The administration of any program, including a pediatric psychology service, can be a lonely enterprise. For this reason, a second important future need is to enhance support and continuing education for the administrative leaders of pediatric psychology programs. For example, administrators may benefit from workshops that focus on common problems that are faced by their programs and strategies to manage them. By sharing strategies that have worked or been proven ineffective in different settings, one can obtain ideas about strategies that may be applicable in one's own setting. Beyond the advantage of generating ideas, the group support inherent in meeting individuals who are grappling with comparable problems may be useful. The continued survival and development of the pediatric psychology programs of the future may well depend on the quality of training and support of administrative leaders.

9

Professional and Ethical Issues in Collaboration

Psychologists who work in medical settings face special dilemmas in maintaining the integrity of their professional ethical standards and autonomy while responsibly managing the demands and responsibilities of consultation with other professions. Psychologists in medical settings are called upon to take into account the traditions and practices of other professional groups with whom they work (APA, 1992). However, this principle does not provide sufficient guidance concerning how one should deal with interprofessional (or interpersonal) differences that arise in collaborative services, teaching, research, or administration. In some instances, interprofessional differences in the application of ethical standards cause tensions between the need to respect the traditions of another profession and the obligation to uphold one's own standards. Most psychologists, even those who have had substantial experience in medical settings, cannot anticipate all of the interprofessional problems that arise. The purpose of this chapter is to describe some of the troubling professional and ethical problems that arise in medical collaborative work in pediatric settings and strategies to manage them.

CONFIDENTIALITY

Confidentiality presents an illustrative set of problems. The obligation to respect the confidentiality of information obtained from other people in the course of their work as psychologists is a primary ethical responsibility of psychologists (APA, 1992). When consulting with colleagues, psychologists are obliged to avoid sharing "confidential information that reasonably could lead to the identification of a patient and share information only to the extent necessary to achieve the purposes of the consultation" (APA 1992, p. 1606). Such standards have been based heavily on professional practice that involves an exclusive relationship between a professional and his or her client, such as in psychotherapy. On the other hand, physicians are quite accustomed to sharing information freely with consultants concerning the details of patient history, diagnosis, and treatment (Belar, 1991). However, the free sharing of information concerning children and their families in medical settings may conflict with psychologists' professional standards concerning confidentiality (Drotar & Sturm, in press). Such problems may be compounded when many professionals have ongoing contacts with a child and family. It is standard operating procedure for medical, nursing, and other staff to share information about a child or family that they deem relevant to the child's care in chart notes and discussion. However, children and families may or may not be aware of such communication. Moreover, depending on the nature of the psychologist's relationship with the child or family member and the nature of information that is provided, such sharing of information could violate ethical standards concerning confidentiality.

In practice, it is often possible to share general information with the pediatrician that is germane to the purpose for which the consultation is made with the consent of the child and family (APA, 1992). In other cases, the psychologist consultant may need to share more detailed or sensitive information with medical staff that concerns the child's feelings or family situation. For example, a psychologist's interview reveals that a child with a chronic condition has problems following his treatment regimen partially because his mother, who is sole caretaker, is depressed and cannot manage this. One could argue that it is important for the child's care that the pediatrician be informed of this issue. However, this mother would certainly be sensitive to information given to her child's pediatrician that could put her in a bad light. Consequently, it is important to clarify limits of confidentiality with the child and family and obtain their consent for information sharing.

In my experience, the informal, rapid-fire nature of information sharing in medical settings can also pose significant problems concerning protection of patients' confidentiality. For example, medical and nursing staff may share concerns about patients in the halls or at the main desk without always noticing that patients or parents may be in earshot. The informal hallway psychological consultation that facilitates rapid, convenient discussion of patient care may also involve public sharing of sensitive information. Moreover, the sharing of detailed information concerning patients' family situations at psychosocial and medical rounds in inpatient or comprehensive care settings may also be problematic. As guests in another profession's setting, psychologists need to take the initiative in informing other professions about their standards of practice concerning confidentiality and about the actions of collaborators that might threaten their ethical standards. Such communication should be handled in such a way that it does not disparage pediatricians' professional practices or impugn colleagues' intentions.

PROFESSIONAL BOUNDARIES IN PATIENT CARE

Psychologists and pediatricians may also have very different perspectives concerning professional roles in patient care. Psychologists have a strict prohibition against maintaining multiple relationships with patients outside of the therapeutic relationship (APA, 1992). On the other hand, some physicians, nurses, or other hospital staff develop social relationships with certain families or children outside of the work situation, e.g. having patients as guests, taking children on outings (Drotar & Sturm, in press, also see Chapter 14). In fact, staff may see such activities as an extension of their role in helping the child and family. Although the psychologist who is consulting with the staff may feel uncomfortable or even distressed by such behaviors, he or she may not have a suitable forum or invitation from their colleagues to comment on them. However, in the event such relationships prove to be distressing in some way to their colleagues or problematic to patient care, the consultant then may have an opening to raise questions. It may also be possible to try to anticipate problems by didactic lectures and discussions of the costs and benefits of various patient–professional relationships.

CONFLICT IN PROFESSIONAL ROLES

As pediatricians and psychologists continue to specialize and develop new areas of professional expertise, there is increasing potential for their encroachment in the professional "territories" of colleagues. For example, a pediatric neuropsychologist may develop expertise in differential diagnosis in neurology and medication management. Pediatricians who have been trained in behavioral pediatrics learn how to provide counseling and parent guidance. Such blurring of professional boundaries can reflect the positive influences of collaborative work. For example, the pediatric endocrinologist who works closely with a psychologist in providing comprehensive care to children with insulin-dependent diabetes mellitus (IDDM) learns practical ways to manage adherence problems. The psychologist who works with her colleague in endocrinology gains knowledge of individualized management of insulin requirements that would be useful in behavioral interventions with children with IDDM and their families.

Although such mutual enhancement of management skills is an important byproduct of effective collaboration, it is not without risks. For example, pediatricians may be annoyed by a psychologist with a special interest in pharmacology who offers suggestions about medications and dosage levels. On the other hand, pediatric psychologists may be quite concerned about the pediatric neurologist who makes informal use of a selected series of psychological tests as a part of his or her assessment. The growing interest of some psychologists in medication prescription privileges suggests that conflicts in professional role boundaries are likely to increase in the future (Barkley, Barclay, Conners, Gadow, Gittelman, Sprague, & Swanson, 1990).

Whether collaborators experience their colleagues' behaviors as infringements on their professional roles depends on the stage and quality of their collaborative relationship among colleagues, their level of communication, and trust. For example, a psychologist who responds to a pediatric colleague's consultation request with "I think this kid is undermedicated" will probably not win friends and influence pediatricians but rather gain a reputation for arrogance. On the other hand, skilled consultants can make suggestions in the spirit of shared problem solving such as the following: "Do you remember that boy we worked with several months ago who was doing poorly and how well he did when his medication was changed? This child looks like he has the same type of problems. We might want to consider a change in his regimen. What do you think?"

INTERPROFESSIONAL TENSIONS AND CONFLICTS IN CLINICAL MANAGEMENT

Differences in professional training, tradition, and philosophies of care can engender conflicts among collaborators. Some of these problems stem from a lack of interprofessional consensus about how clinical problems should be managed. Other problems may reflect differing philosophies about how best to manage more ambiguous aspects of patient care, such as communicating with children and families. For example, many physicians have been trained to limit their disclosure of information and to play a dominant role in decision making about treatment (Katz, 1984). On the other hand, psychologists are generally trained to promote open disclosure of information among children, families, and caregivers as well as involvement of the family and child in medical decision making in accord with their developmental level (Weithorn & Campbell, 1982). If a physician who happens to be a strong proponent of closed communication and authoritarian decision making happens to work with a psychologist who is a strong advocate of a more open, egalitarian approach, conflicts can arise. Clearly, the child and family should not be placed in the middle of such interprofessional conflicts. On the other hand, a psychologist may find in all good professional conscience that he or she cannot accept the physician's views. In some cases, it may be possible to hammer out a compromise or working agreement by discussing the issues, presenting data, and talking to other professionals in the treatment team and to staff in other centers. However, if agreement is not possible, the psychologist and pediatrician may elect to discontinue their relationship in the best interests of their patient.

Another difficult set of collaborative interactions may be generated by parental reactions to a pediatrician's manner or style of communication or treatment approach. Because they spend time with children and families listening to their concerns, it is not uncommon for psychologists or social workers to hear diatribes from irate parents about how particular physicians have managed their care or talked to them or their children. In some cases, parents may have valid points. Problems related to miscommunication are particularly common in teaching hospital settings in which multiple professions have contact with family members. However, it is difficult to know whether and how best to act on these issues. In some cases, it may be sufficient to hear the family out and to help them raise their concerns directly with their physician. In other instances, the psychologist may be able to help physicians understand the source of their conflict with parents.

CONFLICTS IN EXPECTATIONS ABOUT PROFESSIONAL ROLES

Difficult interprofessional conflicts can arise over the role one is asked to take in a clinical or research program. Psychologists are obliged by their ethical standards to avoid participating in activities in which it appears likely that their skills or data will be misused by others (APA, 1992). In my own work, this occurred when I was asked to evaluate children to determine whether they were a good psychological "risk" for renal transplantation. I felt that I could not realistically make such a determination from psychological assessment, nor was it ethical to do so. Eventually, this situation was resolved by the decision to reorganize services for these children and their families and to abandon the search to identify "good candidates" for transplant on the basis of psychological or social data (see Chapter 6).

Consultants may also be placed in limited professional roles by the kinds of activities they are asked to do. For example, my initial requests for psychological consultation concerning infants and young children with FTT focused only on assessment of their cognitive and emotional development. Although these assessments were useful, this role was frustrating because it did not involve treatment. Eventually, it was possible to restructure my role to develop outreach intervention services for this population (Drotar, 1988).

In some situations, interprofessional conflicts reflect a discrepancy or imbalance in what colleagues expect and how they view their collaboration, e.g., one person being satisfied and the other feeling dissatisfied or used. Such tensions are not surprising because collaboration depends on an implicit "contract," understanding, and trust, which may not be clearly or thoroughly articulated (Drotar, 1983). One common source of collaborative discontent is the concern that a colleague is "dumping" patients. Not surprisingly, very difficult patients and time-consuming problems often trigger such concerns. Because physicians are much more likely to refer patients to psychologists (rather than the other way around), psychologists are much more likely to experience such feelings than their pediatric colleagues. Such frustrations are likely to occur when expectations for service are ambiguous and unrealistic, e.g., when a large group of pediatric faculty expect a single psychologist to provide psychological services to *all* their patients.

Other problems may result from colleagues' misunderstanding about expectations concerning the type of clinical involvement that the consultant will assume with patients. For example, a pediatrician refers a patient with a developmental deficit and behavioral problem to a psychologist for an evaluation. Expecting that the psychologist will "handle" the problem, the pediatrician does not set up a follow-up appointment to discuss the results of the evaluation with the child's parents. However, the parents are frustrated because they expected to see the pediatrician, whom they have known a long time, and have a great many questions about the etiology and treatment of their child's problem.

The other side of such collaborative frustration is illustrated by a psychologist who conducts comprehensive psychological testing for a child's learning problem. His test report provides useful information concerning the nature of the child's information-processing deficits but little information concerning remediation. The pediatrician is quite annoyed because the psychologist does not recommend management strategies or offer to help the parents decide about their child's academic placement.

ADDRESSING AND PREVENTING COLLABORATIVE CONFLICTS

Conflicts in collaborative work can create distress and disrupt patient care, teaching, research, and interprofessional relationships. Unfortunately, it is generally very difficult to address these tensions or conflicts for several reasons. Because psychologists and pediatricians have demanding work loads, it is easier to avoid problems than to find the time or muster up the interest to address them. Confrontation and open discussion of collaborative problems are also unpleasant because one runs the risk of hurt feelings. For all these reasons, collaborators may choose to ignore the problem and hope that the situation does not recur. However, although this "ignore and forget" strategy may limit conflict, it does not address the problem.

Consequently, collaborators may need to be more active in resolving conflicts. When trying to resolve conflicts, colleagues should not enter into such discussions when they are angry. Instead, it is important to state clearly (and in a reasonable tone) what the problem is, e.g., "I've been having a problem with . . . that I need your help with" and to emphasize a collaborative goal, i.e., "let's see what we can do to solve this." As in any relationship, placing blame will do little to improve the situation. On the other hand, communicating one's appreciation for a colleague's concession may go along way to reinforce a desired behavior.

Prevention of collaborative conflicts has tremendous advantages over damage control. In general, the more colleagues' expectations concerning collaborative tasks can be clarified, the more effective their work will be. It is rarely possible to clarify, negotiate, and state expectations for all possible activities. However, one can certainly clarify the specific services that will be provided to a pediatrician's patient, teaching expectations (two lectures on hyperactivity, not six), and time commitments, e.g., 20 hours of direct patient contact a week.

Moreover, it is important to anticipate problems that may arise in a future collaboration and clarify expectations accordingly, as in the following example. In meeting with a pediatric GI specialist, a new psychologist, one of only three in a large pediatric teaching hospital, discovers that this specialist would like her to be *the* psychologist for all her patients. In the interests of preserving her sanity and not creating false expectations concerning service availability, the psychologist clearly states that it will not be possible for her to manage the considerable caseload in the pediatric GI service. At the same time, she lets her pediatric colleague know that she is particularly interested in a subgroup of patients, e.g., children with recurrent abdominal pain, and could take such referrals.

PRACTICING WITHIN BOUNDARIES OF PROFESSIONAL COMPETENCE

Psychologists' ethical responsibilities to recognize the boundaries of professional competence and provide services for which they are qualified by training and experience are critical (APA, 1992). In pediatric settings, the ethical dilemmas related to practicing within one's area of professional competence can be intensified by several issues. For example, many pediatricians feel much more comfortable with consultants in their own setting and are very reluctant to refer their patients to "outside" professionals. Moreover, some pediatricians may erroneously perceive any psychologist as an expert on the entire gamut of psychological problems. As one of a small number of psychologists in a particular setting, many pediatric psychologists may be expected to be jacks-of-all-trades and provide assessment and intervention to patients who vary widely in age (infancy through adulthood) and presenting problems. Hence, they may be asked to provide highly specialized interventions for patient groups, e.g., behavioral feeding programs for children with severe feeding disorders, and pain management, e.g., imagery and hypnosis, for children undergoing painful procedures. Even intensive, highly specialized graduate, internship, and postdoctoral training programs simply cannot cover all advances in research and practice in pediatric psychology. For this reason, even very well-trained pediatric psychologists will inevitably encounter clinical and research problems that are new and unfamiliar. After more than 20 years of continuous practice in pediatric psychology, I certainly encounter clinical and research problems that fall beyond my expertise. However, what troubles me is that the number of such problems seems to be increasing exponentially!

In order to be seen as a responsive consultant, psychologists may be tempted to answer as many requests as possible, including some that are clearly outside of their sphere of competence. On the other hand, if psychologists define the zone of their professional competence too tightly, they run the risk of being insufficiently responsive to pediatric colleagues. In fact, it is not always easy to decide whether a particular problem is in one's area of competence or not. For example, should psychologists who have had some experience in assessment of infants on an internship rotation answer such referral requests even though they may not be especially facile with such assessments? At the same time, it is difficult to gain experience with new problems or populations if one does not respond to requests.

LONG-TERM STRATEGIES TO ENHANCE PROFESSIONAL COMPETENCE

Although dilemmas related to boundaries of professional competence are not easily solved, several guidelines may be helpful. Psychologists who are part of a group have several options that are not available to solo practitioners. For example, a psychologist who is not comfortable with his competence with a particular presenting problem should defer to a colleague to see the case or to provide consultation. However, the imbalance between junior and senior-level psychologists in many hospitals may result in a shortage of qualified mentors (Gram, 1992). For these and other reasons, developing consistent structures to enhance professional competence among peers, including peer review and support, may be very important in medical settings (Gram, 1992). For example, regular case reviews can provide a forum for colleagues to discuss difficult cases as well as persistently challenging consultation problems.

Pediatric psychologists may need to develop plans for their continuing professional development that allow them to enhance their professional competence in areas of clinical need that emerge in their setting. In this regard, they should make full use of opportunities for workshops, continuing education, and supervised experience and apprise hospital administrators of the importance of their need for continuing professional education.

However, continuing education is by no means a panacea. One needs to resist the temptation to become an instant expert in a complex area, e.g., deciding one can practice pediatric neuropsychology after completing a workshop. Moreover, it is certainly preferable to focus one's continuing education experiences and patient care experiences to develop specific skills in one or two areas rather than take the professional "smorgasbord" approach.

Sooner or later, almost every psychologist will be requested by pediatric colleagues to practice outside of his or her areas of competence. In such cases, as in other difficult areas of consultation, judicious use of the word "no" is critical (Drotar *et al.*, 1982). The impact of such refusal on pediatric colleagues can be softened by such statements as "I'd really like to help you out, but I've not had much experience with this problem, which really requires someone who is more of a specialist. Let me see if we can find another option." Although such a response may trigger frustration in a pediatric colleague who had his or her heart set on your help, in the long run, it will help colleagues come to trust you.

DEVELOPING AND MAINTAINING PROFESSIONAL AUTONOMY

Professional autonomy is a critical professional need of psychologists in medical settings and is absolutely necessary for optimal program development (see Chapter 8). In many settings, the development of adequate structures to maintain professional autonomy and responsibility for psychologists (e.g., ensuring appropriate supervision for trainees and psychology assistants, credentialing, staff privileges) lags behind the level of development of clinical, teaching, or research programs (Thompson, 1991). In 1984, Thompson and Matarrazo reported that only 13% of the 123 medical schools surveyed had bylaws that enabled psychologists to be full voting members of the medical staffs of their universities. Thompson (1987, 1991) has cogently argued that the development of formal clinical privileges for psychologists in medical settings is critical to the development of professional autonomy in several respects. According to the Joint Commission on Accreditation of Healthcare Organizations (JCAHO), which has been influential in creating a less restrictive medical staff designation in hospitals (Enright, Resnick, Ludwigsen, & Deleon, 1993), hospital privileges constitute the permission to provide medical or other patient care services based on professional license, expertise, competence, ability, and judgments (JCAHO, 1991). The JCAHO requires that there be a single organized staff, e.g., physicians and other licensed individuals permitted by law, to provide patient care services independently that has overall responsibility for the quality of professional services provided by those individuals with clinical privileges (JCAHO, 1991). Bases for membership in the medical staff include evidence of current licensure, training, experience, current competence, and documented experience in specific categories of treatment or procedures. As noted by Thompson (1987), an individual's clinical privileges are hospital-specific and involve a reappraisal for renewal based on current licensure, professional performance, and clinical technical skills as indicated by quality assurance activities and other indicators of continuing professional qualifications such as peer and departmental recommendations.

Beyond the question of delineation of privileges, another important function of the medical staff is quality assurance, which includes implementation of a planned and systematic process for monitoring and evaluating the quality and appropriateness of the care and treatment of patients and clinical performance of individuals with clinical privileges (Thompson, 1991). Physicians can certainly judge whether a psychologist fills the needs of their program, gets along with their staff, and provides prompt service and useful reports. However, pediatricians and hospital administrators cannot adequately judge professional training and experience or delineate standards for privileges and quality assurance for psychologists any more than psychologists can set standards for pediatricians. Hence, pediatric psychologists need to take a leadership role in developing their hospital's procedures regarding clinical privileges and quality assurance, including delineating specific clinical responsibilities for psychologists (e.g., assessment, behavioral therapy) and deciding who is qualified to carry them out. This includes specification of necessary qualifications for general and specific clinical privileges in terms of training, experience, and licensure (Thompson, 1991). Clear delineation of clinical privileges also provides a structure to help ensure that pediatric psychologists practice within the areas of their professional competence.

Enright *et al.* (1993) have noted the importance of ensuring not only that psychology practitioners are recognized as autonomous in hospitals and in insurance plans but also that the broad scope of health-related psychological services is not limited by either insurance plans or hospitals. As noted by Thompson (1991), psychologists should sustain the level of political activism that is necessary to become members of the clinical staff in hospitals and be actively involved in the process of delineating clinical privileges for psychologists. The writing on the wall seems clear enough: if pediatric psychologists do not become actively involved in ensuring adequate standards of accountability for the delivery of their services (as well as research and teaching), eventually someone else will do it for them.

FUTURE DIRECTIONS

The professional issues that have been discussed in this chapter are not the only ones that are encountered by psychologists in pediatric settings. I would hope that this discussion will stimulate others to describe additional "case studies" that illustrate the problematic professional/ethical issues that arise in the practice of consultation and collaboration in pediatric settings. The more that such difficult professional and ethical issues are articulated, the easier it will be to develop guidelines for consultants to consider. It will also be important to gather systematic information concerning hospital and staff privileges, professional autonomy, and responsibilities of psychologists who practice in pediatric settings. Such information will be useful in setting policy as well as in documenting the specific professional issues that need to be addressed in medical settings.

10

Empirical Studies of Consultation and Collaboration

As noted by Roberts (1992), research concerning the efficacy of consultation services is important for the continued development of the field of pediatric psychology. Moreover, data concerning the efficacy of psychological consultation are of great interest to pediatric colleagues who want answers to such pragmatic, "bottom line" questions as whether it helps patients to be referred to psychologists. Empirical studies of consultation and collaboration also have direct practical value for psychologists and pediatricians who want to develop new programs (see Chapter 8). For example, data showing that psychological services are well accepted by hospital staff and parents and make a positive difference in children's lives may help convince key administrators that new programs are necessary. Finally, evaluative research may also help to advance knowledge of the processes involved in consultation and collaboration and thus help to improve the efficiency of methods. The purpose of this chapter is to summarize information concerning physicians', including pediatricians', utilization and perception of psychological services and data concerning efficacy of psychological consultation.

DESCRIPTION OF PSYCHOLOGICAL CONSULTATION SERVICES

Psychological consultation services in different settings have been relatively well described (Drotar, 1976, 1977a; Kanoy & Schroeder, 1985; Ottinger & Roberts, 1980; Singer & Drotar, 1989; Walker, 1979) (see Chapters 3 and 4). The following conclusions can be drawn from such descriptions. (1) The problems seen by pediatric psychologists for clinical consultation vary dramatically as a function of the setting. (2) Pediatric psychologists provide a diverse array of services in response to the needs of populations and pediatric consumers of services. Although assessment is emphasized, interventions, especially brief treatment, are also frequently provided. (3) Following the development of an active, visible consultation service, pediatric psychologists can usually expect a dramatic increase in referrals for service. However, the need to respond to the increasing number of referrals generated by responsive services presents a formidable challenge. (4) Prevention-focused consultation services are not emphasized in most settings unless concerted efforts are made to develop and structure them (see Finney *et al.*, 1991; Schroeder & Mann, 1991, for examples of preventive services).

PHYSICIANS' UTILIZATION OF PSYCHOLOGICAL SERVICES

One set of important but unanswered questions concerns factors that influence pediatrician's referrals of psychosocial problems to psychologists or other professionals. A complex set of actions is required in making psychological referrals. Pediatricians need to recognize a problem as significant, talk to the parent and child about the need for a referral, identify the type of service that is needed, locate a specific referral source, and arrange the referral. In my experience, many pediatricians are very sensitive to parents' attitudes about referrals and weigh them heavily. For example, a survey of general practitioners' referrals to a child psychiatric clinic in Manchester, England, indicated that such factors as parental anxiety (65%), parents' direct requests (59%), and severity of the child's problem (47%) influenced referrals (Bailey & Garralda, 1989). These authors also assessed medical practitioners' expectations from such referrals. The majority (66%) noted that they expected an opinion or advice from the psychiatrist concerning the child's management. However, a sizable percentage also expected treatment of the child (48%), advice to parents (46%), or family therapy (34%). It would be useful to repeat a similar survey concerning pediatricians' referrals to psychologists.

Pruitt, McGowan, Elliot, Koerner, and Mullins (1988) surveyed 248 medical practitioners, internists, family practitioners, and pediatricians to determine obstacles involved in physicians' referrals of patients for psychological or psychiatric services and to determine their satisfaction with consultation. The average referral rate for psychological or psychiatric services by this group was only one per month, which the authors felt represented a small fraction of the potentially referrable cases. However, as a group, physicians reported being relatively comfortable and knowledgeable concerning when to refer a patient for psychological or psychiatric services. Cost to the patient was noted as the biggest obstacle to referral, followed by patient's negative reactions to the referral, lack of knowledge of referral sources, and lack of available referral sources. These data support the influence of situational constraints on referrals (Drotar, 1993).

Pediatric Screening and Identification of Behavioral and Developmental Disorders

One would anticipate that limitations in pediatric identification and screening of behavioral and developmental problems would limit referrals (Simonian, Tarnowski, Stancin, Friman, & Atkins, 1991). In contrast to prevalence rates for psychopathology in ambulatory care settings of 15–20%, the median identification rate of emotional and behavioral dysfunction by pediatricians is 4–7% (Costello, 1986). The reasons for such underestimation are complex but are understandable given the multiple situational constraints on practicing pediatricians, e.g., time pressures, accessibility to mental health resources, difficulty discussing problems with parents (Drotar, 1991, 1993).

In most of these studies, physicians' ratings of behavioral problems have been compared to results of standardized symptom checklists or epidemiologic instruments designed to make specific psychiatric diagnoses. However, this approach may place a difficult if not unrealistic burden on pediatricians who are not trained to diagnose problems in accord with the *DSM* system and often deal with children with subthreshold clinical problems. To address this problem, Horwitz, Leaf, Leventhal, Forsyth, and Speechley (1992) assessed the rates of physician-identified psychosocial problems in a community-based primary care setting using a classification system specifically designed for primary care. This system grouped presenting problems into categories that were much more familiar to pediatricians than *DSM* categories, e.g., physical growth and development (slow weight gain), cognitive/language (language delay), school problems, and family problems (divorce/separation). Pediatricians in this study identified a greater percentage (27.3%) of psychosocial or developmental problems than in previous research. Moreover, pediatricians offered services either directly or by referral to more than half of the patients with problems that they recognized. Factors that enhanced pediatricians' recognition of problems included severity and familiarity with the child (Horwitz *et al.*, 1992). It would be interesting to assess the role of factors such as accessibility of referral sources or level of interdisciplinary collaboration on pediatric identification of psychological problems.

There is also evidence that pediatricians underidentify cognitive/

developmental problems and mental retardation (Goodman & Cecil, 1987). Again, situational constraints involving time pressures, lack of reimbursement for screening, and lack of accessibility of psychological services may contribute to this problem (Feightner & Cadman, 1992). Moreover, screening and early identification of developmental problems involve special concerns about labeling of children as delayed or retarded, problems with validity of screening instruments, and concerns about the efficacy of early intervention (Feightner & Cadman, 1992).

On the other hand, Dobos, Dworkin, and Bernstein's (1994) survey suggests some positive movement in pediatricians' attitudes and clinical approaches concerning developmental problems from 1977 to 1992, at least among a subgroup of 97 board-certified pediatricians. For example, 61% reported that they used a standardized developmental screening test such as the DDST, compared with 38% in the earlier study. The majority (80%), as compared with 38% in 1976–1977, also noted that they made referrals to a psychologist for further evaluation. In fact, nearly 80% of the pediatricians reported that they had at least monthly contacts with psychologists. The source of changes in these pediatricians' approaches is not clear, nor is it clear whether the findings are generalizable.

Pediatric Management of Specific Clinical Problems

Another useful approach is to assess pediatricians' approaches to specific behavioral or developmental problems, where management would logically involve referral to a psychologist. One such problem is attention-deficit hyperactivity disorder (ADHD). Copeland, Wolraich, Lindgren, Milich, and Woolson (1987) summarized pediatricians' ($n = 417$) reports of their practices in the assessment and treatment of attention deficit disorder (ADD). Rather than using specific *DSM-III* criteria for ADD, pediatricians relied on symptoms such as distractibility, overactivity, and impulsivity. Parents were the most frequently mentioned sources of diagnostic information, although history from teachers and psychoeducational reports were also frequently mentioned. Pediatricians reported that they relied on stimulant medication and behavioral modification as treatments of choice. However, parent or teacher behavioral rating scales were utilized by only about 60% of this sample. A large number of respondents (70%) reported employing behavioral modification in the treatment of ADD. However, the nature of and efficacy of this treatment was not clear. Unfortunately, pediatricians' utilization of diagnostic information and treatments provided by psychologists was not described.

Stancin, Christopher, and Coury (1990) surveyed 147 pediatric residents representing a diverse spectrum of training programs ($n = 7$) in Ohio concerning their management of ADHD. The majority of these residents reported that they relied on multiple sources of data, especially history from parents, teachers, physical exams, observation of the child's behavior, parent- or teacher-completed rating scales, and psychological testing. More than two-thirds (69.7%) of the residents reported that they utilized psychological testing "frequently" or "always" in diagnosing ADHD. The majority also reported that they utilized other professionals for evaluation, consultation, or treatment. Residents reported that the professionals they consulted "frequently or always" in the management of ADHD were psychologists (61.8%) and behavioral pediatricians (44.7%). Finally, residents reported that they utilized a range of treatment approaches, e.g., parent guidance, behavioral modification, or counseling for the child, in addition to stimulant medication. The relatively high rates of psychological consultation reported by these residents may reflect the accessibility of psychologists at these teaching institutions. On the other hand, the majority of residents reported practices that suggested continuing needs for collaborative training. For example, the majority (86.1%) used the behavior of the child in the exam room in making the diagnosis of ADHD, whereas only a very small percentage (10%) used objective methods such as rating scales to evaluate the effectiveness of stimulant medication (Stancin *et al.*, 1990). These findings warrant replication at other centers.

Edwards, Mullins, Johnson, and Bernardy (1994) conducted a state-level of survey of general pediatricians' ($n = 116$) diagnostic procedures and management practices concerning recurrent abdominal pain (RAP) in children. Information was also obtained concerning the frequency with which pediatricians encountered children with RAP and made referrals to mental health practitioners and factors that influenced their decisions about consultation or referral. Pediatricians reported that they frequently encountered children with RAP (modal frequency of 2–4 times a month) but referred them much less frequently: 41% made one referral a year or less; 42% made one referral every 2–6 months. The primary management strategies for RAP were reassurance and pediatric follow-up. The low frequency of referrals occurred despite pediatricians' recognition that a relatively high number of children with RAP have chronic symptoms and that psychological and social problems are often associated with RAP. Pediatricians reported that the primary impediments to mental health referral were financial cost, family resistance, and beliefs about the course of the disorder (e.g., likelihood of spontaneous remission) rather than uncertainty about the effectiveness of mental health treatment with the patient group. The authors recommended that integrating mental health practitioners into primary care settings would overcome some of these barriers to referral and allow psychologists to be included earlier in the referral process. Cunningham's experience in managing children with RAP in the context of a collaborative practice with pediatric gastroenterologists (see Chapter 13) supports these authors' recommendation.

PHYSICIANS' PERCEPTIONS OF PSYCHOLOGICAL SERVICES

In accord with the model presented in Chapter 2, pediatricians' expectations of their contacts with a psychologist may influence their utilization of and satisfaction with psychological services and consultation. Several studies have assessed physicians', including pediatricians', perceptions of psychological services. For example, Stabler and Murray (1973) asked pediatricians to indicate which of several services, e.g., testing, therapy, consultation, planning, teaching, provided by pediatric psychologists they viewed as essential. Testing was ranked as essential by more than 90% of the sample, and consultation (90%) and teaching (90%) were also ranked highly. In contrast, therapy (30%) and planning patient care (45%) were rated as essential by a minority of physicians. Stabler and Murray (1973) suggested that pediatricians may perceive pediatric psychologists in a stereotyped way as diagnosticians and hence may overlook their potential contributions in treatment and program development. It would certainly be interesting to repeat this survey today, especially in those settings where pediatricians have been exposed to a full range of psychologists' contributions.

Bergman and Fritz's (1985) national survey of 1,089 fellows of the American Academy of Pediatrics focused primarily on pediatricians' experiences with child psychiatrists. However, this study also provided useful information concerning pediatricians' perceptions of psychologists. The majority of respondents (82%) noted that they had a mental health professional other than a child psychiatrist to whom they referred patients. This group noted that they would regularly refer patients to a psychologist (36%), social worker (10%), or to either a psychologist or social worker (36%) (Bergman & Fritz, 1985). It was interesting to note that 52% of the ambulatory care pediatricians surveyed said that they had either a psychologist or a social worker available in their practice. This high level of perceived availability is somewhat surprising in light of the scarcity of clinical descriptions of psychological services in ambulatory care.

It was noteworthy that pediatricians' preferences for referral sources varied with the clinical problem. Child psychiatrists were the first choice for referrals of childhood depression, psychologists for learning problems, behavioral-oriented pediatricians for hyperactivity (psychologists were ranked second), and social workers for family crises and child abuse and neglect (Bergman & Fritz, 1985). However, some respondents (10–20%) were either unwilling or unable to specify a single preferred professional discipline and noted that they referred to two or more professionals for each of the psychosocial problems, with the exception of depression. It was interesting to note that the majority (77%) of pediatricians believed that other mental health professionals were not as effective as psychiatrists. However, 39% felt that other mental health professionals were more available than psychiatrists (Bergman & Fritz, 1985).

Liese (1986) took a different tack by having residents and staff physicians in different specialties (family practice, internal medicine, and pediatrics) rate the degree to which they felt that interpersonal psychological problems contributed to various medical problems, e.g., depression, alcoholism, obesity, headaches, GI disorders, pulmonary disease, hypertension, and cancer. These physicians were also asked to rate the degree that they expected to be involved in the treatment of these conditions, e.g., noninvolvement to full involvement, and to say which other professions they expected to be involved in treatment of these problems. Physicians ranked conditions such as depression, alcoholism, headaches, and obesity as having strong psychological components. Regardless of their specialty, physicians expressed an interest in treating the psychological components of these conditions and reported that they would consult different professions, e.g., psychiatrists, psychologists, and social workers, on an equal basis. Unfortunately, differences among subspecialists' ratings were not described. It would be interesting to tailor such a survey to pediatricians by asking them to rate the impact of psychological factors on common pediatric problems and their perceptions of the need for consultation from psychologists on such problems.

Physicians' Satisfaction with Psychological Services

How satisfied are physicians with consultations provided by psychologists? Although information concerning this topic is still relatively sketchy, available data indicate mixed results. For example, in the Pruitt *et al.* (1988) survey of medical practitioners that was described earlier, internists were more satisfied with their consultations with psychiatrists than were pediatricians or family practitioners. In contrast, pediatricians were more satisfied with psychologists than internists or family practitioners. However, in the overall sample, psychiatrists were rated as the professional group most likely to be referred to, followed by psychologists, master's-level counselors, and clergy. Internists expressed more dissatisfaction than did the other two specialties with what they perceived as psychologists' lack of medical knowledge and lack of improvement in their patients following psychological intervention. The authors concluded that physicians were not aware of the potential efficacy of behavioral interventions for medical problems such as chronic pain, enuresis, encopresis, etc., as these problems were not likely to be referred.

Meyer *et al.* (1988) surveyed 139 family practice and internal medicine specialists concerning their experiences with psychological consultation for their patients. Physicians were asked about their perception of the competence of psychologists who consulted with them and the utility of consultation. Most respondents viewed psychological consultations as helpful and necessary. However, they also expressed several important concerns about whether psychologists were adequately trained in consultation and sufficiently familiar with medical issues, as well as with the lack of feedback from psychologists during and after referrals for consultation. Moreover, some respondents expressed confusion about how to determine which psychologists were competent.

To my knowledge, there has been no large-scale survey of pediatricians concerning their experiences with psychological consultation. Because available studies have sampled very different practitioner groups using a wide range of methods, it is difficult to draw generalizable conclusions. However, the concerns about psychological services noted by many physicians, coupled with the underutilization of these services, suggest a continuing need for psychologists to demonstrate the need for their service to pediatric practitioners in the community.

Pediatricians' Satisfaction with Psychological Consultation in Specific Settings

An alternative approach to large surveys of physicians in a particular community or region is to assess practitioners' satisfaction with psychological consultation conducted in a particular setting. The survey by Olson *et al.* (1988) of physicians', nurses', and social workers' evaluations of psychological services provided to hospitalized children over a 4½-year period by a pediatric psychology service is unique and particularly instructive. In this setting, the majority of consultations (n = 140) were requested by general pediatricians (40%), surgeons (21%), and adolescent physicians (16%). The evaluation included perceptions of the staff's confidence in their own abilities to identify and treat psychological problems, agreement between staff perceptions of patients' psychological status and feedback from psychologists, overall satisfaction with services, and perceptions of the likelihood of future requests for consultation. A relatively high overall return rate (77 of 170, or 48%) was received. Staff members were relatively confident in their ability to identify patients in need of psychological services but less so in their ability to provide psychological services. Presumably this increased the likelihood of referral.

On the whole, the respondents reported a high level of satisfaction (3.6 on a five-point scale ranging from 1, not at all to 5, very) with overall services. The psychology service also received consistently high ratings from staff on various dimensions such as timeliness, usefulness, quality of feedback, and effectiveness of intervention. In addition, respondents reported a high probability that they would request services in the future and a high likelihood of a significant negative impact in the event psychological services were to be discontinued. Such data clearly indicate a high level of staff respect for this particular pediatric psychology service. The staff reported the lowest overall satisfaction rating (equivalent to a "somewhat satisfied" rating) concerning the psychologists' outpatient follow-up of the hospitalized children. The majority of respondents (67%) felt that patients seen for inpatient consultation should be followed as outpatients by pediatric psychology. This service had in fact provided outpatient care for nearly a third of the patients, but the referring staff may not have been aware of this.

Level of staff satisfaction with consultation was highly related to the level of mutual diagnostic agreement, which was generally high, between the referring individual and the pediatric psychologist's feedback concerning the child. Because of the potential importance of the agreement variable in this study, it would be useful to determine the factors that contributed to level of agreement and disagreement among consultants and referring professions.

Acceptability of Psychological Services

To my knowledge, there have been few if any studies of the degree to which pediatricians regard specific recommendations made by pediatric psychologists as acceptable and/or whether they actually follow them. Tarnowski, Kelly, and Mendlowicz (1987) used an interesting methodology to assess nurses' perceptions of psychological interventions that is applicable to physicians. Pediatric nurses were asked to review one of six written case vignettes that represented two levels of behavioral problems (mild tantrums versus aggression causing damage to property) and several levels of medical problem severity (severe = leukemia, mild = anemia). Case descriptions were followed by a series of six interventions that were grouped into conceptual categories, such as accelerative, e.g., praise, parent-mediated reinforcement, token economy, versus reductive, e.g., systematic ignoring, response cost, time-out procedures. Each of these interventions was described as having one of three levels of time involvement ranging from minimal (less than 10 minutes per day) to maximum (1 hour per day). Interventions applied to severe behavioral problems were rated as more acceptable than those applied to mild behavioral problems. However, medical severity did not make a difference. Methods involving more positive reinforcement methods were generally rated more acceptable than techniques such as time out. Respondents preferred parental reinforcement and response cost procedures that involved moderate time commitments. Clearly, additional work is needed concerning physicians' ratings of the acceptability of psychological interventions.

EVALUATION OF PSYCHOLOGICAL SERVICES IN PRIMARY CARE SETTINGS

The central question for the pediatric and family consumers of psychological services concerns the efficacy of these services. Randomized controlled trials of the efficacy of psychological consultations cannot be conducted because it is not ethical to withhold services from clients. However, it is possible to conduct descriptive evaluations of services, and several such studies have been reported in primary care settings. For example, Kanoy and Schroeder (1985) addressed the following questions in their report. (1) Can short-term, cost-effective intervention be offered in a pediatric primary health care setting? (2) What are the most effective suggestions for behavioral and developmental problems raised by parents? (3) Do parental concerns continue to exist at the time of follow-up? The sample included all parents (60% of those who were eligible) who participated in follow-up evaluations from 1973 to 1980 for the following concerns about their children: toileting ($n = 54$), sleep ($n = 60$), developmental delays ($n = 21$), negative behaviors ($n = 60$), sibling/peer difficulties ($n = 49$), and personality/emotional problems ($n = 38$). Follow-up evaluations were done between 2 months and 2 years after the original contact, with most of the contacts being made within 1 year. Parents were asked to rate on a 1 (low) to 5 (high) point scale the effectiveness of each suggestion that had been made, the general services, and the counselors who provided them. Parents were also asked if they had any current concerns about their child's behavior and development. In general, parents evaluated the psychological service and counselors quite highly. With the exception of developmental delays, in every area of concern, at least 88% of parents rated the service as good. Parents rated the suggestions for socialization and behavioral problems higher than for developmental problems. Finally, the relatively high percentage of parents who expressed concerns (40–80% for many categories) on follow-up underscored the necessity for additional follow-up studies.

Charlop *et al.* (1987) assessed the efficacy of behavioral management of 100 children who were referred to a pediatric psychology service at a university-based center, the Kennedy Institute at Johns Hopkins University. The majority of these children were from low-SES families. The intervention involved parent training that included general guidelines and specific strategies to rectify targeted problem behaviors, e.g., modeling of prescribed behavioral solutions by therapists, opportunities for parents to imitate the therapist followed by feedback, written protocols summarizing recommendations, and child-rearing texts. Instructions were also provided to parents concerning observing and recording target behaviors and, in some instances, coordination of home-based behavioral management with academic and behavioral performance in school. Parents were encouraged to keep weekly parent training appointments. However, intervals between appointments were gradually lengthened when improvement in the child's behavior was noted. Most cases involved 4–12 treatment sessions over a 1- to 6-month period.

Evaluation included information from medical records and a brief (15-minute) phone contact with parents at 3, 6, and 12 months posttermination. Information was obtained concerning occurrence of the child's presenting problem behaviors, parental utilization of strategies that were recommended, and whether the parents continued to employ recommended strategies. Parents rated whether the frequency target of behaviors had decreased, increased, or stayed the same, whether new problems had developed, and how they were addressing them. Finally, parents rated their level of satisfaction with the parent-training services they received on a five-point scale (1, extremely dissatisfied to 5, extremely satisfied).

Parents generally reported improvement in their children's problem behaviors from the intervention to the point of termination. Moreover, additional improvements or maintenance of treatment effects were observed for most problem behaviors from termination to the 3- to 6-month follow-up. By the 12-month follow-up point, the frequency of some target behaviors had increased, but others remained below termination levels.

Among children who were initially seen as inpatients and then provided services, improvement, defined as decreases in frequency of target behaviors by 20% or more compared with baseline, was noted in 73.7% of cases. No apparent change was noted in 26.3% of cases. Among outpatients, improvement was noted in 80% of cases with no change or an increase in frequency of problem behaviors in 17.3% and 2.7% of cases, respectively.

Across the entire sample, an impressive 70% of all parents reported that no new behavior problems had occurred since the termination of services. Moreover, the majority (67%) of parents were judged to select appropriate strategies and hence to generalize what they had learned in order to manage new behaviors. Finally, the vast majority of parents reported satisfaction with recommendations: 30.3% were very satisfied, 50.2% satisfied, 9.2% somewhat satisfied, and only 1.3% reported that they were extremely dissatisfied. Parents noted the qualities of the therapist, the practicality and efficacy of treatment recommendations, availability, and emphasis on positive reinforcement as factors relating to their satisfaction.

Charlop *et al.* (1987) felt that these positive treatment outcomes were somewhat surprising because almost half of the cases were considered by the therapist to have terminated prior to the attainment of agreed-upon treatment goals. These authors also noted the persistence of some behavioral problems at point of follow-up and hence the need for longer-term follow-up.

Another important question concerns the extent to which pediatric psychology services can reduce the level of pediatric health care utilization. To address this question, Finney *et al.* (1991) evaluated a psychological consultation service that was established by a department of pediatrics in a health maintenance organization that served middle-class families. The service model involved brief targeted therapy in which parents and their children were typically seen in 50-minute appointments from one to six times (mean 2.4 visits) for common behavioral and emotional problems. Parents were helped to define specific problems, and treatment goals focused on changes in the targeted behaviors. Parent behavioral management methods were prescribed for specific problems such as reinforcement for appropriate behavior, time out or ignoring for undesired behavior, positive practice and retention control, and reinforcement, e.g., for toileting problems, contingency contracts, e.g., for school problems, and self-management and parental reinforcement, e.g., for chronic pain. To ensure adequate implementation of recommended therapeutic techniques and to manage problems that arose, most families also received a number of planned telephone contacts.

Research assistants who had not been involved in clinical services contacted parents of treated children at 3 or 5 months following termination of treatment. Parents rated outcomes of their children's problem from "completely resolved" to "worse" and completed a short form of the Child Behavior Checklist (Achenbach, 1991) and ratings of satisfaction with services (1, dissatisfied to 5, very satisfied). Therapists also completed ratings of the child's outcome, and information was obtained from the child's medical records concerning the number and type of visits and diagnostic problems of medical visits.

The majority of parents (76%) reported that their children's problems were resolved (30%) or improved (40%), whereas a smaller number of parents reported problems to be unchanged (20%) or worse (4%). Therapists' outcome ratings agreed with 80% of the parent ratings. On follow-up, parents were generally satisfied with treatment, with 49% reporting that they were very satisfied, 33% satisfied, 11% somewhat satisfied, and only 6% unsatisfied. Following treatment, parents also described positive changes in their children's symptoms. One of the most important findings was a significant decrease in the treated group's medical encounters from a mean of 8.76 visits per person year before treatment to 6.34 visits after treatment. This reduction of apparently excessive visits was most prominent for children who presented with behavioral problems and toileting symptoms as compared with school and psychosomatic problems. Use of medical services was unchanged during the same time period for a matched comparison group of children from the practice.

This is one of few studies to demonstrate an "offset" effect, that is, the reduction in medical care use after mental health treatment, among children. The findings suggest that psychological treatment may reduce parents' tendency to seek out medical care in order to have a health care provider respond to their distress (Finney *et al.*, 1991). Finney, Lemanek, Cataldo, Katz, & Fuqua (1989) demonstrated a similar decrease in utilization of medical care as well as an improvement of pain-related symptoms among children with recurrent abdominal pain (n = 16) who received a multicomponent target therapy that included self-monitoring, limited parental attention to symptoms, relaxation training, and school attendance.

FUTURE DIRECTIONS

Taken together, the studies reviewed in this chapter provide preliminary evidence of the efficacy of psychological consultation services in pediatric settings. However, there is a continuing need for follow-up studies of children who have received psychological services. It would also be useful to assess factors that influence pediatric utilization of psychological services in accord with the model of collaborative activity presented in Chapter 2. Another important direction for future research concerns the assessment of psychologists' roles in enhancing clinically relevant outcomes, e.g., quality of patient–provider outcomes, including adherence and appointment keeping (see Chapter 3).

[illegible]

11

Training Psychologists in Consultation and Collaboration

The number of specialized training experiences in pediatric psychology at graduate, internship, and postdoctoral levels has increased in recent years (Davidson, 1988; LaGreca, Stone, Maddux, & Drotar, 1988). However, there is no clear consensus on basic training objectives and content (Mesibov, 1984) and substantial variation in how these programs achieve their aims. It may be more difficult to design programs to train psychologists to consult or collaborate with pediatricians because these are inherently more ambiguous tasks than other clinical activities. Moreover, various characteristics of pediatric hospital settings, e.g., hectic clinical pace and limited structures for interdisciplinary communication, can limit effective teaching of collaboration. Consequently, clinical supervision of pediatric psychologists tends to focus much more on assessment and management of various pediatric problems than on methods of consultation or collaboration. Consultation issues tend to be discussed incidently, such as in response to a "problem" with a particular pediatric resident or faculty member. Moreover, supervisors may assume that trainees will automatically acquire skills in consultation in the course of their clinical training. However, this "implicit learning" approach to training in consultation is problematic. In the absence of supervised discussion of consultation issues, trainees may not learn to recognize common consultation dilemmas or develop strategies to manage them and may never come to appreciate their strengths and weaknesses as consultants.

In contrast, supervised discussion and didactic work expose students to a tradition of consultation methods and theory (Caplan & Caplan, 1993). The importance of collaboration in the professional functioning of pediatric psychologists and the development of pediatric psychology programs argues for its formal and systematic inclusion in professional training. For example, Stabler and Whitt (1980) recommended that the pediatric psychologist be trained to work within a "practitioner–consultant–scientist model" as opposed to the more standard "practitioner–scientist model". However, the central goals of training in psychological consultation and methods of such training are not well articulated. The purpose of this chapter is to describe issues and strategies in training psychologists to work with pediatricians.

FACILITATING A CONTEXT FOR TEACHING COLLABORATION

There are many possible models of training psychologists to conduct consultation with pediatricians (Davidson, 1988; Stabler & Whitt, 1980). In the course of providing clinical and research training to graduate students in pediatric psychology, my colleagues and I have used a range of approaches that have been adapted to the setting and content of training activity that have been guided by several basic principles. One is that students benefit from observation of psychologist–pediatrician collaboration at a faculty level. A second principle is that students should have an opportunity to practice skills in collaborative research, clinical work, or teaching under supervision. Another is that the benefits of such observational and practical experiences are enhanced by didactic lectures that discuss empirical data concerning consultation and collaboration.

In my experience, students will not have a successful training experience in consultation unless the faculty has paved the way by creating respect for psychology among pediatric colleagues and a professional context in which the student can be supported and trained among a network of collaborators. In my setting, I did not conduct training until I developed a sufficient referral base, the presence of psychology in the setting, and structures for interdisciplinary collaboration (Drotar, 1976, 1977a). To accommodate students at different levels, I have utilized several different models including a 3-month rotation in pediatric psychology as part of an clinical child psychology internship, a year-long placement for advanced (third-year and beyond) graduate students, and a 1-year postdoctoral training experience. Although it was possible to provide useful training in each of these models, I believe that the more intensive models, i.e., a year-long practicum or postdoctoral training, were more effective because they provided a better fit with the setting. In my experience, a more continuous experience is needed for students to develop their own collaborative relationships with staff and to obtain sufficient exposure to setting problems and characteristics. The varied consultation issues that present in inpatient or primary care settings means that training experiences should be tailored to these settings.

TRAINING IN INPATIENT CONSULTATION

In the inpatient setting, observation of hospital rounds and consultations and direct supervision of students' consultations proved to be useful teaching methods.

Supervised Observations of Hospital Rounds

We have found it helpful to have trainees observe collaborative case-review meetings that focused on the psychosocial aspects of care and were attended by members of various disciplines (Drotar, 1978). These meetings provided an excellent opportunity for students to observe physicians' and nursing staff's confrontation of psychosocial problems related to their work setting. For example, common problems on the young adult unit included management of noncompliant adolescents, psychological support of chronically and terminally ill patients, and the management of adolescents in the midst of psychological crisis (Drotar, 1977b). This gave students a first-hand appreciation of the work-related dilemmas of physicians and nurses, particularly the impact of the hectic, crisis-oriented work pace on their interactions with families.

Regularly scheduled supervisory meetings provided opportunities to discuss students' observations on the rounds and to discuss the content and strategy of the meetings (see Chapter 4). Students have been struck by the heavy emotional burdens encountered by pediatricians and nurses in their daily work. In my experience, many were also surprised by pediatricians' limited training in psychosocial aspects of care. Some were unduly critical of physicians' limitations. Supervisory discussions also allowed clarification of students' feelings about the medical and nursing staff and encouraged empathy for the staff's roles. Readings that described the culture of medical settings (Fox, 1957) and consultation methods (Caplan, 1970) were also useful.

Observations of Informal Contacts

Students' learning of consultation can be facilitated by borrowing from the medical model and having them tag along to observe the supervising psychologist interact with physicians, nurses, social workers, child life staff, etc. An action-oriented consultant who is very visible in making frequent rounds and has a busy consultation service provides a model to students as well as an engaging, "live" learning experience. Students learn most effectively if they can discuss their observations and ask their supervisor "Why did you do that?" "What did you think Dr. X meant by that?"

Clinical Supervision

Clinical supervision of student case consultation is a basic training method. For beginning students it is most helpful if the supervisor takes an active role in structuring the consultation, e.g., by finding out relevant information from the referring pediatrician and helping the student identify the consultation question. More advanced trainees can eventually take a more independent role by assuming responsibility for all contacts with staff. I have found that cases that involve the student in an active role in intervention, e.g., providing support for an anxious hospitalized child while working together with multiple hospital staff, can be particularly gratifying.

To maximize students' learning from case consultation, some of the supervisory time should be devoted to discussion of general consultation issues using case material. For example, a request from the resident for help with an overanxious child and parent can be used to discuss issues including any concerns the resident had about the child and family? What was the resident's role with the child and family? Was he or she comfortable with it? How can the information from the psychological evaluation be used to facilitate the resident's role? The opportunity to engage in discussion with pediatric residents who are also in training can enhance students' comfort with pediatricians and understanding of how they approach clinical problems, constraints on their time, etc. Pediatric residents and fellows derive similar benefits from their contact with psychology trainees.

My experiences have consistently supported the need to teach students how best to communicate with hospital staff, e.g., the need to communicate clearly and in a highly practical manner, the need to review the hospital chart thoroughly, and the importance of clearly documenting notes in the chart and adapting psychological methods to fit the demands of the setting.

TRAINING FOR CONSULTATION IN PRIMARY CARE

Primary care settings also provide very useful experiences and training contexts for psychologists to learn consultation (Kanoy & Schroeder,

1985). One such training experience takes place in the Continuity Care Clinics in the Department of Pediatrics at MetroHealth Medical Center in Cleveland, where pediatric residents also receive training in primary care (T. Stancin, personal communication, Dec. 14, 1993) (see Chapter 3). Since 1987, graduate students, typically third-year students in the pediatric psychology program at Case Western Reserve University, have participated. As part of a clinical practicum experience, they are assigned to a particular clinic afternoon and become an integral member of the clinical team. Training experiences have typically included three core elements. These are: (1) observations of pediatric providers including well-child appointments, administrations of immunizations and medical procedures, child life activities, e.g., medical play, and precepting activities that are conducted by a pediatrician, psychologist, and/or nurse practitioner; (2) participation in team meetings, including responsibility for presenting one topic during the year; and (3) consultation and direct service. Under supervision, a trainee provides service to selected team patients, who typically have such problems as attention deficit disorder with hyperactivity, in evaluation of childhood adjustment problems, parent training, etc.

This training experience has several significant benefits for students. Students are exposed to a role model of a psychologist who is actively engaged in interdisciplinary teaching and clinical activities and to an opportunity to participate as a member of a team. As one recent trainee stated:

> I was able to work in a group setting . . . not just interdisciplinary, but truly collaborative . . . it was such a benefit to work in a situation where people from different professions were comfortable working in tandem. This countered the impression I had that physicians and psychologists don't get along. With the right people and structure, there is good outcome for both.

Based on their experiences, student trainees learn to appreciate the multiple demands that are placed on pediatricians in providing primary care to children, as noted by this student's response:

> Rather than reading in a textbook or journal article about how primary care in pediatrics operates, I am having the opportunity to view it first hand. This makes me better able to imagine what process a client has gone through before being referred to me for psychological services. I am gaining a real appreciation for the time pressure on residents and physicians to see many patients in a short time period. I never thought before that the 50-minute hour psychologists spend with patients is actually a luxury!

One of the important features of this experience involves the opportunity for trainees to see a broad spectrum of children including those with essentially normal psychological development as well as children with emerging psychological difficulties. Such broad exposure is generally not available to psychology students whose experiences are often limited to children who have already been identified as having serious behavior and developmental problems. Because families often seek advice from their physician when they are most motivated to seek help for their children, trainees can begin working with them immediately, unencumbered by the lengthy referral/waiting-list process that is more common in traditional mental health settings. As one student noted, "I have been able to see a patient referred directly from a physician and to see that patient in the clinic setting. This has been useful to make the referral process much more real for me. I am understanding more about how problems get detected and how physicians decide to make referrals to psychology."

Students also have an opportunity to receive training in rapid consultation under close supervision such as in the following example. A psychology trainee accompanied a second-year pediatric resident who saw a 12-year-old boy for a well-child visit. This was the first time this child was seen at this hospital; the family lost private health insurance coverage when the father became unemployed. The child's mother presented concerns that had been raised by the child's teacher regarding his poor school performance, lack of concentration, poor attention, trouble following instructions, and mildly disruptive behavior. The child had been placed on methylphenidate (Ritalin) by his previous physician, but that was discontinued because of side effects such as "dizziness." The child stated that he has "trouble understanding what is going on" in class. The child's pediatric exam and a review of medical history were unremarkable. Together the psychology student and resident reviewed their impressions with the staff psychologist, who agreed that records should be obtained from the boy's previous physician and from the child's teacher. Behavior rating scales, including the Child Behavior Checklist (Achenbach, 1991), were given to the child's parents and sent to his teacher for completion. An appointment was given to the family for the following week to see the psychology trainee for a more detailed clinical interview, to review school records and behavior rating scales, and to determine what additional information or psychological testing might be indicated. The psychology trainee then worked together with the resident and psychologist and pediatric preceptors as a team in making additional treatment recommendations (T. Stancin, personal communication, Dec. 14, 1993).

COMMON DILEMMAS FOR STUDENT TRAINEES

Trainees experience several common dilemmas in their collaborative work with pediatricians. For example, trainees' zeal concerning their newfound consultation skills and acumen can sometimes threaten pediatric colleagues. As a psychology intern, I remember proudly communicating my findings concerning my evaluation of a child with somatic symptoms and school avoidance and a strong recommendation for psychotherapy to the referring pediatric resident, who was managing the child's care. I was both dismayed and angered when what I saw as my cogent findings and recommendation were not exactly met with open arms. Not wanting to upset the family by recommending psychotherapy, the resident responded with: "Primum non nocere" (do no harm). I remember thinking, how could *my* recommendations do harm? Expecting the resident to accept my pearls of wisdom without question, I was quite frustrated by the experience. However, in retrospect, I did not adequately consider what the resident wanted to find out from the consultation.

Trainees often have unrealistic expectations concerning pediatricians' knowledge base and abilities to manage children's behavioral and developmental problems. Dialogues with supervisors and pediatric colleagues can help trainees develop appropriate expectations of their pediatric colleagues. One goal of supervision is to help students steer a difficult line between expecting too much of pediatric colleagues and becoming frustrated and expecting too little. When I first started working with pediatricians, I was not as aware of the limitations of pediatric training and the stresses on pediatric residents as I am now. I expected pediatricians to make highly specific referrals, to be "sensitive" to the nuances of interactions with their patients, and to be eagerly interested in my teaching. With experience, I have learned to be more tolerant of pediatricians at all levels, especially those in training.

Some students also have difficulty being sufficiently assertive and directive in their consultation work. It is very easy for students to be intimidated by physicians' authority, especially in unfamiliar medical settings. As a trainee and as a junior psychologist, I was much more tentative in interactions with physicians than I am now. In my supervisory sessions with students, I have emphasized the need for them to make assertive (rather than tentative) recommendations to pediatricians and to help pediatric colleagues arrange necessary case dispositions.

Students also need to learn to set priorities in their consultation and to communicate basic information clearly to pediatricians, nurses, and other staff in face-to-face contacts and written notes. This is not easy to do because most students are not aware of the information that pediatricians find most useful. Psychology students' appreciation of consultation issues can be enhanced considerably by supervised experiences in giving teaching conferences to pediatric residents. In this way students have a "trial by fire" in preparing a lecture to pediatricians, identifying information that is most useful to them, and fielding their questions.

Veteran pediatric psychologists are accustomed (though, ideally, not inured) to witnessing the painful experiences and distress of children during pediatric hospitalization and surgery and working with children who have been disfigured and with highly stressed families who have multiple problems. Many trainees who confront such experiences for the first time are understandably distressed by them. For this reason, they may need additional support and opportunity to discuss their emotional reactions.

TRAINING FOR COLLABORATIVE RESEARCH

The graduate-level Pediatric Psychology Research Training Program at Case Western Reserve University has the primary goal of training psychologists to conduct research and practice with pediatric populations (Drotar, 1991). To enhance this aim, our program has implemented several strategies of teaching and promoting students' interest in collaborative research.

Exposure to Models of Pediatric Practitioners and Researchers

One important ingredient of this training is to involve graduate students with pediatric researchers and practitioners and hence expose them to pediatric thinking about clinical and research problems. Students participate with fellows in the behavioral pediatrics training program in a teaching seminar that is coordinated by a psychologist and a social worker. This involves presentations by various professionals, e.g., social work, pediatrics, psychology, anthropology, child psychiatry, in their areas of expertise. Pediatricians with specific interests in common behavioral problems, e.g., sleep or feeding problems, impart the wisdom of their considerable clinical experience and thinking about these problems to students. In this way, students learn to appreciate the full range of behavior problems that present to pediatricians as well as interventions that are possible in pediatric practice. Seminar discussions also include the benefits and problems of the interdisciplinary clinical care. Students' participation in this seminar has the added benefit of facilitating their contact with pediatric residents who have similar interests in behavior and development

Didactic Training

Students' appreciation of the expertise and contribution of pediatricians has been enhanced by pediatric faculty members' lectures in their area of specialty that cover the basics of pathogenesis and treatment of pediatric conditions, e.g., cystic fibrosis, cancer, neurological disorders.

Students hear pediatricians' views of the essentials of clinical management of frequently occurring conditions and address such questions as: What psychological problems are associated with particular pediatric conditions? What does the pediatrician want most from a psychologist who works with this population? What problems has the pediatrician encountered in working with psychologists?

Pediatricians can also provide models of scientific practitioners who have managed to conduct successful research programs in behavioral and developmental pediatrics while managing to fulfill strenuous clinical and teaching responsibilities. In didactic lectures, students hear pediatricians' perspectives on the development and implementation of their research in such areas as the effects of iron deficiency on behavior (Lozoff, Jimenez, & Wolf, 1991) or the impact of a socially supportive companion during labor (Kennell, Klaus, McGrath, Robertson, & Hinkley, 1991).

Wherever possible, we have also tried to expose students to models of successful pediatrician–psychologist collaboration. Presenters have included pediatricians, psychologists, and social workers who had worked together in providing comprehensive family-centered care for children with mental retardation and chronic physical problems and research teams involving psychologists and pediatricians.

Collaborative Mentorship and Research Teams

In some instances, pediatricians have provided mentorship for graduate students to learn specific research skills, e.g., working with observational data, physiological measurement of response to stress. In other cases, students have joined interdisciplinary research teams that have been organized by pediatric faculty. Such training opportunities have been a particularly valuable component of students' research clerkship experiences. For example, one student, Karen Berkoff, became particularly interested in the pediatric residency as a model for work-related stress. In her research clerkship, she teamed up with Wayne Rusin, a member of the pediatric faculty who had similar research interests, who worked with her on a pilot study of house officers. Their collaboration led to the development of a master's thesis on the effects of the stresses of call duty on residents' distress (Berkoff & Rusin, 1991) and to dissertation research on the effects of resident gender and personality style on their health behaviors and psychological status (Berkoff & Drotar, 1994). Pediatric faculty, Rusin and Lozoff, participated in Berkoff's master's and dissertation research committees and provided helpful feedback and support. Thus, students receive the benefit of feedback and conjoint mentorship from a pediatrician and psychologist.

Ongoing collaborative research among psychologists and pediatricians in our setting has also provided a fertile context for students to obtain research-related experience. For example, another student, Yonit Hoffman, joined a research team headed by John Kennell, a pediatrician, and Sue McGrath, a psychologist, on a study of the effects of a supportive companion (*doula*) during labor on outcome of labor and delivery, e.g., incidence of cesarean section. For her dissertation research, Hoffman (1992) worked very closely with this research team studying the impact of the presence of the *doula* on maternal psychological adjustment, e.g., mood, self-esteem.

Facilitating Student Research through Collaboration

For many years, collaboration with pediatricians in our setting has also facilitated students' master's- and dissertation-level research studies involving a wide range of pediatric populations, especially children with chronic physical illness (e.g., cystic fibrosis, diabetes, sickle cell disease, asthma, and cancer) (Bull & Drotar, 1991; Kucia *et al.*, 1979; Moise *et al.*, 1987) and high-risk infants (Singer & Fagan, 1984; Phipps & Drotar, 1990). Pediatricians and nurses have played a valuable role in this research by facilitating recruitment of children and families, giving advice concerning research design, and sometimes serving on students' master's and dissertation research committees. In a recent and exotic example, an interdisciplinary research project concerning the impact of HIV infection on Ugandan infants (see Chapter 7) provided a context for several students (Drotar, Peterson, & Berkoff, 1992) to conduct pilot research on determining the applicability of cognitive tests (Bayley Scales and Fagan Test) to Ugandan infants. Subsequently, one of these students, Nancy Peterson, then developed and conducted her dissertation research concerning the effects of maternal HIV infection on Ugandan infants' security of attachment (Peterson, 1994).

I have found that students' experience in research-related collaboration facilitates their learning of generic lessons. For example, collaborative research commonly raises interprofessional differences in opinions about research design, measurement, and definitions of "good" or relevant research (Drotar, 1989). Such issues can facilitate useful discussions of differences in psychologists' versus pediatricians' perceptions of research, approaches to research design, and ways to reconcile or manage these difficulties (see Chapter 7).

Students can learn a great deal from the tensions created in the course of collaboration so long as they have support and backup from a supervisor who can and will intervene on behalf of the student if necessary. This type of collaborative research training also requires the talents of students who are willing and able to assume a high level of independence in their scholarly activities and are sufficiently confident to stand their ground in the heat of collaborative differences.

Effective collaborative research training requires trust on the part of pediatric colleagues that the student will be competent and productive. This type of trust is not automatic but is gradually built up over years based on successful faculty-level collaboration and pediatricians' direct experiences with students. A successful collaboration with a student will leave pediatricians wanting to repeat this experience and hence more research opportunities than one can fulfill. On the other hand, a negative experience with a student who does not meet faculty expectations will shut down opportunities. In this regard, it is very important that students compulsively follow up with pediatric colleagues in all phases of their research, especially by communicating the results of the research to the staff and the families who participated.

TRAINING AND SUPPORT FOR FACULTY

Faculty psychologists typically regard students as the ones who are in the role of learners in consultation activities. However, I have been impressed with the wide range of difficult professional and ethical issues that are raised by consultation that tax even the most seasoned consultants (see Chapter 9). For this reason, pediatric psychologists need to develop ways to obtain support and continuing education for their consultation and collaborative ventures. Several avenues are possible. For example, experienced consultants need opportunities for feedback and reality checks with colleagues to consider questions such as the following: Were they too harsh in setting a limit on a pediatrician's unrealistic request? Were they sufficiently clear in giving feedback to a pediatric colleague about problematic interactions with parents? Many of these consultation problems do not have quick and ready solutions or right answers but involve a difficult set of cost-versus-benefit decisions about consultation strategy. Such discussions of collaborative work also provide a mechanism of mutual support and planning for programs (see Chapter 8).

Support for Collaborative Teaching at a Regional Level

One of the more interesting models of faculty support for training in collaborative teaching was developed by the Behavioral Pediatrics Consortium of Northeastern Ohio (Stancin *et al.*, 1989). This consortium was developed by the coordinators of behavioral pediatrics training at three northeastern Ohio residency programs to promote collegial support, collaborative educational programs, professional development, and program evaluation. It has since expanded to include more than a dozen faculty members and several behavioral pediatric fellows at six pediatric residency programs. Although this consortium was developed to promote training of pediatricians rather than psychologists, the structure of this group can facilitate the training of many professionals.

Collegial Support. Perhaps the most important function of this group has been to provide collegial support, e.g., a forum for group problem solving, and to obtain consultation about programmatic issues. The informal, collegial atmosphere of the consortium has enhanced group sharing and support.

Collaborative Educational Programming. At each meeting, the group discusses ideas for educational programming. Curricula at each residency program have been shared, aspects of various programs have been adopted at different sites, bibliographies of educational resources have been developed, and new teaching references and resources have been identified. Members are encouraged to be invited speakers at other sites, thus maximizing the available resources for a teaching pool. Plans have been made to sponsor an annual regional continuing educational conference involving consortium members and visiting scholars as faculty.

Professional Development. One of the most important features of this group is its interdisciplinary composition, which includes psychologists, social workers, developmental and behavioral pediatricians, and a child psychiatrist. Consortium members can identify with others of the same profession who work in similar roles at different sites and collaborate with those of different educational backgrounds who are struggling with common concerns. Moreover, junior faculty who may have had limited access to role models within their own institutions can benefit from the experiences of the more senior members of the consortium. Senior members, feeling the strain of years of isolation, have felt reenergized by the enthusiasm and struggles of junior members (Stancin *et al.*, 1989).

Program Evaluation and Collaborative Research. Collaborative evaluation strategies, such as site visiting, peer review of programs, and uniform evaluation procedures, have been utilized. This consortium has conducted collaborative research projects in areas of mutual interest such as a study of residents' strategies of evaluating children with attention deficit hyperactivity disorder (Stancin *et al.*, 1990).

FUTURE DIRECTIONS

There is also a need to provide continuing education for psychologists who are involved in training psychologists to consult with pediatricians. Experiences concerning training in collaboration and consultation can and should be shared in written descriptions. Pediatric psychologists should continue to share their experiences in training students in consultation and collaboration at local and national meetings. Descriptions of innovative methods of training psychologists to provide consultation to pediatricians and other professions would be particularly instructive, especially if accompanied by data concerning the outcome and activities of former students.

Part II

New Opportunities for Collaboration with Physicians

INTRODUCTION

I wanted this volume to strike a balance between my review and synthesis of writing on collaboration and consultation, largely with pediatricians, and descriptions of new opportunities, especially with other physician groups. Hence, I invited several colleagues to contribute descriptions of consultation and collaboration with physicians in various settings and with different populations. Each of these authors has provided readers with an interesting, first-hand look at the collaborative issues that arise in various settings.

First, Hurley (Chapter 12) takes the reader step by step through the practical, "nuts-and-bolts" issues involved in starting a pediatric psychology practice. Her description of the negotiation process with pediatricians, including legal and contractual issues, is particularly instructive.

Cunningham (Chapter 13) follows with a useful report of her collaborative practice with pediatric gastroenterologists. To my knowledge, this is the first published description of a psychologist's collaborative practice with a pediatric subspecialty.

Rosenthal's (Chapter 14) description of consultation in an adolescent medicine training setting documents psychologist–physician collaboration in a broad range of clinical service, research, and training activities. This report is noteworthy for its description of interdisciplinary collaborative tensions concerning supervision and teaching.

Finally, Crawford (Chapter 15) describes issues and opportunities in psychological consultation with family practitioners who see large numbers of children and families in primary care settings. Crawford's description illustrates the important but underexploited opportunities for collaborative teaching and intervention with this specialty.

Taken together, these contributions illustrate the kind of diversity in collaboration that will be needed if psychologists are to meet the challenges of the 1990s, which include ensuring that greater numbers of children and their families have access to psychological services in increasingly diverse settings (see Chapter 17). I would hope that this work will stimulate others to contribute descriptions of their consultation and collaborative activities. To discuss similarities and differences in the experiences of these consultants and to integrate the information that is presented in this section, these four chapters are followed by a brief summary of issues and implications.

12

Developing a Collaborative Pediatric Psychology Practice in a Pediatric Primary Care Setting

LINDA K. HURLEY

The practice of pediatric psychology within a primary care setting is not a new idea (Schroeder & Mann, 1991). However, such collaborative practice is by no means widespread, and most psychologists are not found practicing in the typical pediatrician's office. Schroeder (1993) found that only a handful of psychologists identified themselves as having a full-time practice within a pediatric primary care setting.

The impetus for me to approach some pediatric groups in Fort Worth, Texas came from informal discussions with two other psychologists who had similar practices. Carolyn Schroeder had begun a part-time training program in North Carolina for psychologists and pediatricians within a primary care clinic approximately 18 years earlier. This effort was initially funded in part by grant money and was focused on training and research as well as clinical work. In that way, it was quite different from what was available to me in my community. Mary Evers-Szostak had developed a practice with a pediatric group in Durham, North Carolina, which was closer to the prospects that were available to me (Evers-Szostak, Schroeder, & McClure, 1991).

LINDA K. HURLEY, Ph.D. • Fort Worth Pediatric Clinic, 851 West Terrell Avenue, Fort Worth, Texas 76104.

Before considering the possibility of joining a pediatric group, I had considered joining a group of psychologists for private practice. At the time, there was only one other pediatric psychologist in independent practice in Fort Worth. However, she worked with a group of psychologists and did a combination of pediatric, child, clinical, and adult psychotherapy. Several other child psychologists were practicing independently or within agencies or the school system. I had been warned that a pediatric psychology practice would not be viable in Fort Worth, but it appeared that joining a psychology group would necessitate expanding my practice to adolescents and adults, which I neither desired nor felt competent to do.

I had previously consulted with local pediatric gastroenterologists, who seemed generally pleased with and supportive of my work. Moreover, they expressed some frustration that pediatric psychology services were not readily available to them, since there were no psychologists on staff at the local children's hospital. As a result of their interest, I approached the local children's hospital (Cook-Fort Worth Children's Medical Center, CFWCMC) to encourage them to develop a pediatric psychology division and offered my services. I developed a formal proposal and presented it to the medical director of the hospital. He expressed some interest in the idea but left the decision up to the new psychiatrist, who felt that no psychologists were needed within the hospital. This decision was frustrating because it was apparent (to me) that there was a need for pediatric psychology. However, not everyone shared my perception nor recognized pediatric psychology as a legitimate subspecialty. In communities where pediatric psychology is better established, one has the opposite challenge: making a niche for oneself where others have already carved up a significant portion of the available pie. However, I did not have the option of locating elsewhere, as I was married to a Fort Worth native who had a well-established dental practice and had no intention of moving anywhere. Since I genuinely wanted to develop this type of practice and had nowhere else to try, I approached several pediatric groups in Fort Worth and was eventually successful.

SETTING UP A PRACTICE

Clinic Location and Structure

Fort Worth Pediatric Clinic (FWPC) is located in a free-standing building that is owned by the two senior partners in a joint venture. The building is located in the medical district of Fort Worth, Texas, and is approximately six blocks from CFWCMC. Several other major hospitals primarily serving adults are also located within approximately a 2-mile radius from the clinic, as are a number of physician practices.

The staff of FWPC consists of four M.D. pediatricians, seven full-time nurses, six part-time nurses, and 10 office staff. The ages of the physicians range from 34 to 42 years. There are approximately 20,000 patients in the practice. The clinic currently operates as most private pediatric practices in this area do, with office hours 9–5 on weekdays and emergencies seen after hours and on weekends as needed.

Negotiating with a Pediatric Group

Unless they have trained with pediatric psychologists, pediatricians generally have only a vague understanding of psychologists and what we do. In my experience, most have no idea of such issues as the length of assessment or treatment session, how many patients we see per day, problems that are seen, fees and reimbursement, how long treatment takes, whether our tests are valid or reliable, etc. Although physicians may *believe* they know a great deal about psychology and psychologists, much of their "knowledge" may be outdated, invalid, based on assumption rather than fact, or simply untrue. For example, pediatricians may assume that a psychology practice is the same as a pediatric practice. One must keep this basic lack of information in mind in approaching pediatricians to discuss collaborative practice. Therefore, the most important step after establishing contact with a potential collaborator(s) is to determine what he or she knows or believes about a psychologist's professional role and activities and to correct and fill in gaps in that knowledge, preferably with concrete data.

In April, 1991, I approached the four pediatricians in the FWPC with the idea of contracting space and two other group practices in the area. I initially sent each physician in each group a letter stating that this was a useful opportunity for them to add to their practice in a very practical way, that my services were reimbursable by third parties, and that I had some experience with pediatric offices and how they operate. I also pointed out my unique strengths, enclosed a copy of my vita, and stated that I would call them to arrange an opportunity to meet with them.

My philosophy is that one should approach negotiations with pediatricians with an attitude of cooperation, clearly emphasizing that the new service would enhance both pediatric and psychology practices. In such negotiations, it is essential to have the practice plan well thought out. I used the strategy of presenting this plan verbally, accompanied by handouts to take home. This not only allowed an opportunity for discussion but also provided the pediatricians with something to take with them to stimulate additional thought. I presented a three-page summary of what services had been offered by other pediatric psychology practices, what advantages could be anticipated, along with reprints of articles about pediatric psychology.

Following these presentations, the responses of two of the three groups were negative. The other group, FWPC, expressed interest and was willing to set up an additional appointment for me. However, the FWPC physicians were mixed in their responses. Two of the doctors were more interested, while the others were more reluctant. One of their concerns was that FWPC would be responsible for keeping me busy with referrals. This concern was lessened by the agreement that I would solicit referrals from a number of different sources and would assume responsibility for all aspects of my practice. The physicians were then more willing to structure the agreement as a sole proprietorship rather than as a clinic employee, which was also my desire. In addition, the pediatricians from FWPC called the pediatricians at Durham (North Carolina) Pediatrics, with Dr. Evers-Szostak's office, to get additional information on how their practice had incorporated a psychologist, and on their (very positive) impressions of this arrangement.

Space was another significant issue during these early negotiations. The clinic was at capacity and had even added offices in an attic to provide additional room. There appeared to be no space that would be suitable for a professional office. However, at this point, the physicians were seriously interested in adding this service and hence were more willing to try to accommodate my needs. After examining every square foot of office space, we agreed that the billings and collections specialist could be moved into a smaller but more private office upstairs and that I could take her current office, which was actually designed as an X-ray room. This space was quite small, measuring 8½ by 11 feet, with a storage area and sink that measured approximately 6 feet by 8½ feet. Although the space was considerably less than desirable, it was agreed on because it was actually the only space large enough and private enough to serve in the present building. Moreover, there was no possibility of adding on. I also felt that it was preferable to take a tiny space in a practice where a psychologist was seen as a positive addition, rather than taking a larger space in a less compatible practice.

Pediatric Psychology Practice Structure: Legal and Accounting Issues

After completing negotiations over a 6-month period, it was agreed that I would be a sole proprietorship and would contract with FWPC for space and services. A set fee was established for office space rent and for specified services, including billings and collections, office reception, telephone, copying, and other standard office services and supplies. All supplies (e.g., test materials) specific to the psychology practice would be my responsibility.

In our contract, it was clearly stated that FWPC had no responsibility to refer patients to me, and no fee would be paid for referrals. At the suggestion of the certified public accountant (CPA) and the attorney who developed the contract, several other contractual points were included primarily to establish the independence of the two practices. I strongly recommend that anyone beginning a practice such as this consult with both an attorney and a CPA before agreeing on anything. Although one may incur substantial costs for this consultation, in the long run the savings and peace of mind are well worth it.

Although I had no business experience, I had the advantage of being married to a dentist who had been in private practice for 15 years. He was most helpful in avoiding the pitfalls of owning and operating a small business. All too often, psychologists forget that operating a private practice is the same as opening a new business, and it should be treated as such. It is clearly helpful to have a friend or spouse in private practice who can mentor you through the start-up process.

Consultation with an attorney was also critical in clarifying several other issues. In Texas, as in most states, it is illegal for a Professional Association (P.A.) to have mixed professions as associates. In other words, a group of psychologists cannot have a psychiatrist as an associate, although it is legal to hire another professional as an employee. In order to establish and maintain the independence of two practices sharing space and personnel to the IRS and others, one must be cautious in how a contract is written.

Meeting with a certified public accountant is also important to help identify and manage the costs associated with independent practice. For example, a significant amount of self-employment tax is calculated in addition to income tax. If this is not paid according to the IRS rules, penalties and interest will accrue, and the amount owed will be significantly more than the already significant amount.

When you are self-employed, all benefits become your responsibility, such as health insurance, retirement, and so on; however, the number of legitimate deductions also increases. A CPA can help you keep records so that you can claim all the legal deductions to which you are entitled at the end of the year. If you do not consult a CPA until tax time, you may miss a significant number of deductions.

Most individuals opening a private practice will also need to establish a relationship with a banker and will probably need a loan to cover start-up expenses. Your bank can explain the types of loans you qualify for and the terms. Your CPA can guide you in selecting the most appropriate type.

DEVELOPING THE PRACTICE

Services

As a rule, I spend approximately 45–50% of my time doing assessments or assessment-related tasks (scoring, interpreting, dictating), 25% doing therapy (individual or parent training), and the remainder doing administrative tasks and telephone calls. On entering private practice, I had no idea of the sheer variety of patient concerns I would encounter. Many of the referral questions related to adjustment and developmental issues—e.g., adjustment to divorce, parental imprisonment, new siblings, moving—and to problems related to sleep, eating, toileting, and other normal issues of childhood. I also had a significant number of referrals for ADHD, emotional problems, negative behaviors, and school problems (Schroeder & Mann, 1991).

Reimbursement and Expenses

Being a provider for health maintenance organizations (HMOs) frequently means accepting a lower reimbursement rate than one's normal charges. In addition, HMOs require additional paperwork as well as justification of the need for services. Because reviewers are often not well trained, the psychologist needs to educate and explain the need for his or her services. The importance of being a provider for HMOs appears to vary from city to city. In some locations, HMOs are rarely used to pay for health/mental health care, whereas in others, they are the standard. Becoming a provider for several major HMOs has been a benefit to me because most people in my community pay for their health care with their insurance rather than out of pocket. As a provider for the major HMOs operating in this area, I not only was able to accept the patients referred from within the pediatric group but was referred a significant number of other patients by the health plans. The physicians in my group felt that becoming a provider for the primary HMOs used by their patients was essential to making the collaborative practice work. If I were not a provider, patients from within the practice would need to be referred out to another psychologist, which would have defeated the purpose of having a psychologist on site.

Marketing

A practice obviously cannot succeed if no one knows about it. Despite the fact that my four associates referred to me, I needed to do a great deal of marketing to build my practice, particularly since I had assured them that they would not be responsible for keeping me busy. Marketing can be done in several ways. One of the best ways is simply to be very visible and to familiarize the staff with your name and services. During the early days of my practice, when I had virtually no patients to see, I still spent every day in the office so the nurses and doctors would see me and remember to refer to me. This also allowed me plenty of time to chat with the nurses and get to know office staff, so they would be better able to talk to patients about me and to know what kinds of things I could do. I consider this informal marketing.

I sent announcements of my practice opening to all the physicians on the staff of the local children's hospital and to all the psychologists and psychiatrists in town. The cost of the announcements and postage was less than $600, which would have been paid for by a single referral for an evaluation. Before having them printed, I asked each associate at FWPC to review the format and make comments. Their comments helped me to design an announcement that was appealing to physicians and would give the information they most wanted. I included a brief summary of my training and experience and a list of available services.

As summer approached and both the physicians and I became less busy, I continued to market my practice by taking lunch to some other pediatric practices and giving an informal presentation about my practice. I generally included both nurses and doctors in these meetings, since nurses seem to make as many referrals as doctors.

Marketing can also be done by including articles in the local newspaper or newsletters. One must be careful in doing this, however, as some advertising of this type is unprofessional. Being interviewed by the local paper for an article is a better choice, especially if the reporter does a good job and accurately quotes or paraphrases your interview. Giving talks to local parent groups or associations sometimes generates referrals, but in my experience this has not generated many. Attending meetings of the local psychological or pediatric association or similar groups can be beneficial, particularly if the pediatricians you work with introduce you and praise you to their colleagues. It often helps for physicians to have met you before they suggest to their own patients that they come to see you. Sending inexpensive holiday gifts and cards is another way of generating referrals and reminding people of your practice.

Becoming involved in one's professional community is also very important to develop a practice. Serving as an officer in your local or state psychological or mental health association can be very helpful in this regard. When patients call a psychologist who does not work with children or on the particular problem presented, he or she is more likely to refer to someone familiar.

Research

Maintaining a successful private practice is a full-time job. In fact, most independent practitioners work far more than 40 hours per week. However, much of the time I spend working is not reimbursable or is reimbursed at a rate lower than my advertised charges because of HMOs and other factors. The only way I am paid is by seeing patients and having the patient or a third party pay for it. Given the demands of the setting and the absence of available student colleagues, research has generally not been possible, with the exception of research that is closely tied to the practice, e.g., assessing parent perceptions of services.

Developing Referrals

My practice has evolved extremely rapidly. Initially, I anticipated being busy for a few days per week and that it would take several months to a year or two to become busy on a full-time basis. To the surprise of everyone, this was not the case. The first month was quite slow as furniture, stationery, test supplies, and a number of other things needed to be ordered and set up. However, within a few months, there was a 2- to 4-week wait for an appointment. Now, after 2 years, there is a 2- to 4-month wait during the school year. The first year, business was very unpredictable, but it has since become more steady.

The FWPC physicians referred a number of patients from within the practice. Several outside referrals were also received, but at first, the bulk of referrals (about 60%) came from the physicians or their nurses. It seemed that simply having a psychologist visible and available in the office stimulated the idea of making a referral. After 2 years, this initial trend has been reversed: approximately 40% of referrals are from within FWPC, and 60% come from elsewhere.

In addition to referrals, several consultations were generated per week. These consisted of nurses asking me about a particular patient and trying to decide whether a particular type of problem was worthy of a formal referral. Physicians also asked for consults, either by stopping by my office or dropping off a chart and note asking to be consulted later in the day. Initially, developing the psychology practice was a matter of educating the staff as to what a psychologist can and cannot do. Most of the questions asked were actually appropriate referrals, often in the form of "do you do X?" or "would you see a patient with X problem?" The opportunity to inform colleagues what a psychologist could do about a specific problem generated even more referrals of similar problems. Although the physicians were very interested in having a psychologist available, the nurses actually did much of the footwork in getting patients referred. Having the nurses as allies has proven to be a great help in facilitating patients actually getting to the psychologist (see Chapter 5). After a patient is seen or has been called on the telephone, giving immediate feedback to the referring pediatrician is essential. In the context of a practice, such feedback can be quite informal but is expected and appreciated.

As other pediatricians and pediatric subspecialists in town became aware of the pediatric psychology services at FWPC, outside referrals increased. The FWPC physicians were quite helpful in introducing me to colleagues at meetings and other events and encouraged their colleagues to make referrals. Interestingly, one concern expressed by the physicians prior to agreeing to have a psychologist in the practice was that of outside referrals. Although the pediatricians did not want to be responsible for keeping me busy, they were also concerned about the perception of other pediatricians that they were "stealing" or "wooing away" their patients. This has not been a problem. Patients referred from other practices are always referred back to their primary care physician for follow-up care, and in-house follow-up is offered only to established patients in the practice.

Parents' Perceptions of the Practice

In the summer of 1993, approximately 20 months after I joined the pediatric group, a pilot survey of parent perceptions was conducted. A second wave of the survey was completed in October, 1993, at two sites: one by Dr. Evers-Szostak in Durham, North Carolina, and one in Fort Worth, Texas (Hurley, McIntire, & Evers-Szostak, 1994). To find out what the parents thought about having a pediatric psychologist in the pediatric group, a survey was designed and administered. This was done partly to encourage other pediatric psychologists to consider collaborative practice arrangements and to be sure our perception that we were being well received by parents was correct.

The results of the survey indicated that 66% of parents knew about the psychologist, and 12% had actually had some interaction with her. Of those who had not interacted with the psychologist, 69% listed "not needed" as the reason. Twenty-two percent indicated they did not know about the service. Although callers frequently ask for evening or weekend appointments, which are not offered, none of the respondents stated they had not used the service because of the hours available. The majority (94%) indicated they thought having a pediatric psychologist in the pediatric office was an excellent (65%) or good (29%) idea. Only 6% rated it as "neutral," and no one thought it was a bad or terrible idea. Some parents expressed concerns about confidentiality with the front office (5%) or the pediatricians (6%), and about feeling pressured to use the psychologist in the practice (11.5%) rather than someone else. However, most (76%) saw no major disadvantages of having a psychologist in the pediatric practice. On the contrary, 85% felt their children would be more comfortable in a familiar setting, and 63% felt that parents would be more comfortable in a familiar setting. They also thought that communication between psychologist and pediatrician would be enhanced by this arrangement (79%).

We also collected demographic data and information on what additional services, e.g., parent groups, parents would like the psychologist to offer. These will be used to build additional services into the practice. The total cost to do this survey was about $400 to $500 per site plus 12 hours of time. A clerk was paid for data entry, and the statistician agreed to coauthorship in exchange for his work.

OUTSIDE CONTRACTS

One drawback of a private practice is financial insecurity. One never knows from month to month what one's collections will be, and whether the bills can be paid. In order to manage this potential problem and to stimulate collaboration within the hospital, I decided to approach the director of the hematology–oncology service directly to propose a contract with his clinic.

A formal presentation was made to the head of the department and to the staff oncologist, stating what pediatric psychology could provide for the clinic and giving a rough time estimate for each service. This allowed the physicians to see how many hours would be needed to do the work they requested. There was a history in this particular clinic of the physicians becoming disgruntled with a psychologist who promised more than he could deliver in the amount of time allotted. Providing a realistic list of psychological services and their time requirements gave physicians a better idea of how to utilize my time. In addition to the time estimates, a suggested priority list was included to help the oncologist decide what they should request initially. If additional funds were available, or the contract was expanded to additional hours, they could request additional services. This seemed to help frame the contract in a way that was acceptable to all.

In addition to the contract with hematology–oncology, an additional contract for psychological services was continued with the craniofacial deformities clinic at the local public hospital, John Peter Smith Hospital (JPS). The chief of oral surgery and I negotiated this arrangement independent of the hospital administration. This contract was initially started when I was employed at a local agency and has continued.

ISSUES AND CHALLENGES

Simply starting a pediatric psychology practice within a primary care setting is a challenge, particularly when there are no model practices available locally for primary care providers to evaluate. It was fortunate, in this case, that a group of pediatricians were willing to take a slight risk on a new practice idea. As stated before, the two other large practices in town were also approached and turned down the idea without any further consideration. Interestingly, these three practices have now agreed to merge. I will stay with the new group as the pediatric psychologist, with the consent of all of the physicians. The larger practice will certainly present challenges that are not evident yet. The number of physicians will be increased from four to 13 full-time pediatricians, with attendant increases in nurses and office staff. This will present a difficult challenge in getting to know each other and to know the individual styles of each person.

One disappointment has been the relative unwillingness of the pediatricians to include me in the merger meetings during which decisions regarding the new practice are made. I have not been directly involved in decisions about such issues as what computer system to use, who the office manager will be, and so on. However, issues may be overlooked that may directly affect my practice. Since I expressed these concerns to the pediatricians at FWPC, they have become somewhat better at informing me of the outcomes of their meetings.

Ongoing Communication

Communication is always a challenge in a busy practice. In other practices, I am told that the doctors meet regularly to chat and catch up on activities, and the psychologist is generally included in meetings with staff or physicians. This has not been the case at FWPC. I begin seeing patients before the pediatricians finish rounds or arrive at the office. The office lunch hour is normally late (1:00 or 1:15) and runs into my afternoon appointments, so lunch has not been a good time to visit except for a brief "hello" in the lunch room. Many of the doctors' meetings are scheduled after work. Despite requests to be included, I have not been invited.

Expanding the Practice

Adding additional psychologists to the practice would help lighten the work load. However, as noted earlier, the current building is at capacity. Thanks to the merger, this will be changing in a few years when all three pediatric groups move into a larger space. The current plan is that the psychologists will have their own space, which will be designed to their specifications. In the meanwhile, one of the merger groups has offered to lease space and services in their office to a second psychologist. Negotiations are under way to hire another Ph.D. licensed psychologist.

Another challenge will be to get the second psychologist to become a provider on the same HMOs and to educate the new doctors and staff on how and when to make referrals. Thus far, the major HMOs in the community have refused to allow another provider which presents the dilemma of how to use a second psychologist.

Implications for Training in Collaborative Practice

My graduate training was in clinical psychology with an emphasis on child practice, and my internship was in pediatric psychology at a medical school. Those aspects of my training that were most relevant to developing the type of practice described here, included a good understanding of child development and developmental issues and the experience of observing and working closely with pediatricians and other health care providers. Having the opportunity to view children and families from a different profession's point of view enabled me to communicate more effectively with others as well as to respect the unique contributions each discipline has to offer in the complete care of the child. My interdisciplinary training in a university-affiliated program (UAP) also proved to be a wonderful opportunity to work with physicians. Finally, my collaborative experiences with pediatricians while working at different jobs were also very helpful in increasing my comfort with pediatricians' needs for rapid feedback and practical suggestions and in providing me with contacts in the pediatric community.

Most graduate psychology programs do not train their graduates to be small business owners. Approaching a private practice with the attitude that practicing psychology is all you want to do will not work. You must manage a business, and to do that successfully requires business knowledge. It is, therefore, necessary for anyone entering private practice to learn about running a business. This can be accomplished by independent study, college courses, relevant readings, or a variety of other training opportunities.

MANAGING THE FUTURE CHALLENGES OF PRACTICE

My practice has been forced to evolve in response to the business decisions made by the FWPC physicians. They have made these decisions largely in anticipation of health care reform, believing there will be strength in numbers in negotiating contracts with third-party payors. My independence from the group means that I may not benefit the same ways they will. Many psychologists in this area are making similar moves by joining coalitions to negotiate for mental health care contracts. I continue to exercise this option, joining mental health negotiating groups while maintaining my independent status.

As this is written, I continue to face unanticipated challenges. The pediatric merger has already cost me a significant amount of money, about which I was neither consulted nor given much notice. Decisions that affect my practice are often afterthoughts to the pediatricians who are trying to run their practices while dealing with their own challenges. This has served to underline the extreme importance of effective and frequent communication between psychologists and pediatricians.

I have found that I need to develop and maintain regular communication with professional colleagues to maintain my own mental health and to avoid professional and personal isolation. This can be accomplished by scheduling regular lunch dates with other professionals, attending meetings, and establishing professional groups such as journal clubs or peer supervision groups.

Although the office practice of pediatric psychology in primary care settings has had some trouble catching on with pediatricians in many parts of the country, my experience suggests that as more and more physicians and psychologists become aware of the potential success of this model, it will become more common. In my setting, both parents' and physicians' perceptions of pediatric psychology in primary care have been overwhelmingly positive. From my vantage point, the advantages of private practice in this setting (e.g., independence) far outweigh the disadvantages. However, you must work hard to make things run smoothly. In the end, a successful private pediatric psychology practice will be the reward.

13

Collaborative Psychological Practice in Pediatric Gastroenterology

Clinical Issues and Professional Opportunities

CARIN CUNNINGHAM

In response to emergent clinical needs and advances in medical treatment of pediatric problems, pediatric psychologists have developed clinical consultation programs that are tailored to individual settings and pediatric specialty groups, including comprehensive clinical care to children with chronic conditions (Koocher, Sourkes, & Keane, 1979). For the most part, such descriptions of collaborative psychological consultation and comprehensive care have been restricted to programs in large tertiary care pediatric hospitals. However, children with chronic conditions may benefit from comprehensive medical and psychological services provided in their communities. One such population is children with gastrointestinal (GI) disorders. Pediatric gastroenterologists in local communities provide medical care to children with a wide range of chronic conditions, including inflammatory bowel disease (IBD), Crohn's disease, ulcerative colitis, ulcers, and encopresis, many of whom have extraordinary needs for psychological services (Whitehead & Schuster, 1985). Pediatric gastroenterology is an ideal specialty for such collaborative practice for several reasons. The numbers of pediatricians being trained in this specialty afford improved

---

CARIN CUNNINGHAM, Ph.D. • Department of Pediatrics, The Mt. Sinai Medical Center, One Mt. Sinai Drive, Cleveland, Ohio 44106-4198.

accessibility to psychologists. Even more important, clinical management of problems seen by these specialists requires a comprehensive interdisciplinary approach that is very difficult if not impossible to achieve by professionals working in isolation (Gillman, 1994). However, to my knowledge, the psychologist's role in the office practice of pediatric gastroenterology has not been reported but offers significant collaborative opportunities that are described in this chapter.

A COLLABORATIVE PRACTICE MODEL

Evolution of the Practice

The present practice evolved over several years of collaboration that began during my postdoctoral training. A group of pediatric gastroenterologists at a tertiary care children's hospital wanted to have a psychologist learn about their specialty and work closely with them in providing clinical services. Recognizing that psychological factors contributed to many clinical problems and needed to be addressed in their clinical management, these specialists were interested in psychological services that were tailored to their patients' needs and closely coordinated with medical care.

The combination of strong physician interest in psychological services, particularly on the part of the chief of this specialty, and the compelling clinical problems presented by these patients and their families presented an excellent training opportunity. As a part of my postdoctoral training at Rainbow Babies & Children's Hospital in Cleveland, I was assigned to work with these specialists and provide psychological services to their patients. During a 2-year experience, I gained a good working knowledge of the symptoms, treatment, and natural course of pediatric GI disorders, the impact of these problems on families, and the interplay between these children's medical problems and their psychological functioning. Moreover, these pediatric specialists felt that their patient care had improved as a result of the increased availability of psychological services. When they left the academic setting to form a private practice, they invited me to join them.

Description of the Practice

The private practice that evolved now consists of three full-time pediatric gastroenterologists and one Ph.D. clinical psychologist and has been in operation for 6 years. For 2 years, I was supported by funds generated from patient fees and a small grant ($6,000 per year) from the hospital to describe parental coping with pediatric and adolescent IBD. The fees that I generate are received by the practice. Overhead for my office space is paid out of these fees. In turn, I receive a salary, funds for travel to professional meetings, supplies, and malpractice insurance. Approximately 80% of patients in this practice are from middle- and upper-class families and have some form of insurance coverage. The director of the practice and I meet to discuss clinical and administrative issues whenever necessary. A yearly meeting is also held to review progress and discuss salary adjustments.

SUMMARY OF CLINICAL SERVICES

In order to obtain information concerning the kind of psychological consultation that was provided in this new practice, I reviewed the psychological services during three separate 6-month periods covering a span of 5 years. Although referral patterns had been quite consistent, there was a significant increase in the total number of patients referred in each of the 6-month periods over a 5-year period, from 55 to 94. The two most common medical presentations were functional encopresis and recurrent abdominal pain (RAP). The type of patient referrals remained constant with the exception of a decrease in the referrals of ulcer disease patients from nine to one. The most common referral problems have included noncompliance with medical treatment plans, possible depression, toileting problems, behavioral problems, school avoidance, family conflicts, and pediatric feeding problems. Psychological services most typically employed have included psychological testing, individual psychotherapy, behavior modification plans, parent guidance, and, in some instances, school consultation.

PSYCHOLOGICAL CONSULTATION FOR SPECIFIC MEDICAL PROBLEMS

Psychological consultation in a collaborative pediatric specialty practice such as ours raises special issues related to collaborative management of clinical problems. These issues reflect the special challenges involved in coordinating clinical care of children with chronic psychophysiological problems who are frequently seen in this practice (see Chapter 6 for a discussion of these issues). Consultation issues have been highly intertwined with the specialized clinical problems seen in our practice. For this reason, frequently occurring problems and relevant management strategies are summarized briefly to orient readers to these issues.

Inflammatory Bowel Disease

Inflammatory bowel disease (IBD) subsumes the related problems of Crohn's disease and ulcerative colitis (Kirsner & Shorter, 1982), which are usually diagnosed among older adolescents and young adults. Prior to diagnosis, symptoms such as anorexia, weight loss, abdominal pain, fatigue, and lethargy were generally confusing and stressful to children, adolescents, and their families. Following diagnosis, families had to cope with the chronic stressors of treatment regimens including medications that, in some instances, affected the child's physical appearance, physical growth, and mood swings (Whitehead & Schuster, 1985). Referrals of IBD patients ($n = 15$) have typically occurred at predictable points in the course of illness management, e.g., at time of diagnosis, recurrence of symptoms, or around specific problems such as noncompliance. Psychological intervention with newly diagnosed patients has focused on helping the child and family accept and manage their symptoms such as diarrhea and pain as well as the extraordinary demands of immediate care such as nasogastric tubes, not being allowed to eat for long periods of time, and diagnostic procedures such as multiple X rays.

Other children and adolescents were referred after a recurrence of their IBD required hospitalization and stimulated intense feelings of depression, frustration, and fear. Most of these children and adolescents became less distressed following collaborative intervention including time-limited supportive psychotherapy during hospitalization and close outpatient follow-up with their physicians.

Noncompliance with medications, particularly corticosteroids, was the third major reason for referral of IBD patients. Immediately following diagnosis, their adherence with all aspects of the IBD treatment regimen was generally acceptable. Most children and adolescents were relieved to be feeling better and to have a medical explanation for their symptoms. However, as the months wore on, many patients became increasingly noncompliant when they no longer felt sick, were put on a lower medication dosage, became aware of medication side effects, and were increasingly frustrated with diet and activity restrictions. To avoid side effects such as cushingoid features, weight gain, acne, and mood swings, some adolescents took themselves off their prescribed medicine, lowered the dosage, or medicated themselves in response to symptoms such as bleeding. Such problems were understandably very frustrating to their physicians, who were reassured by my interventions that focused on helping their patients improve their adherence to treatment regimens.

Encopresis

The largest single group of patients who were referred ($n = 77$) were those with encopresis. The treatment approach to encopresis in our practice followed a collaborative model similar to that described by others (Walker, Milling, & Bonner, 1988).

Ulcer Disease

Pediatric ulcer disease patients were typically referred for psychological evaluation to address physicians' concerns that emotional stresses might be affecting the course of the child's illness (Whitehead & Schuster, 1985). In such cases, we have found it particularly helpful to identify the salient stressors and the coping strategies that were used by children and their families to manage their disease. Moreover, individual psychotherapy and relaxation therapy have also been helpful to some children and adolescents.

Recurrent Abdominal Pain

A relatively large number of children, adolescents, and young adults ($n = 70$) with recurrent abdominal pain (RAP) were referred for psychological evaluation when the degree or type of their pain was not consistent with physical findings and/or when the child had associated problems such as school avoidance or depressive symptoms. Intervention strategies for RAP have been based on a comprehensive evaluation that included the child's developmental history, the family's medical/psychological history, assessment of the relationship between pain complaints and life stresses, and evaluation of possible depression. Intervention with this patient group required very close communication between my physician colleagues and me in comprehensive management plans that emphasized reduction of the child's secondary gain for symptoms, involvement of the parents, especially the mother, in psychological treatment, and in some cases, individual psychotherapy and/or stress management with the child.

Colitis

Children and adolescents with mild colitis ($n = 23$) who were referred for psychological help often had physical symptoms that resembled those of RAP patients as well as accompanying problems such as school avoidance that also required collaborative management and very close communication between the physicians and me.

Feeding Problems

Patients ($n = 30$) were also referred for feeding problems and associated symptoms such as failure to thrive. Many of these children had physical problems such as esophagitis that began in early infancy and made eating quite painful. Despite improvement in the child's physical status, some of these feeding problems persisted and became quite stressful to parents. A subgroup of children was referred because of sudden, dramatic refusals to swallow solid foods, which were associated with traumatic experiences surrounding the act of swallowing.

As reported by others (Iwata, Riordan, Wohl, & Finney, 1982), we found behavioral treatment of feeding problems to be helpful. However, close medical follow-up was also critical to help parents of these children maintain a demanding behavioral program and address their fears about the impact of these eating disturbances on their children's physical health.

COLLABORATIVE PRACTICE ISSUES

All of the clinical management problems encountered in our patients reflected a close interrelationship between medical and psychological factors. Consequently, we decided to provide psychological services as an integral part of the day-to-day care of pediatric GI patients and their families rather than as a separate adjunct to medical care. To develop such highly coordinated care, which is very difficult to accomplish in practice, we have implemented various methods of collaborative problem solving, consultation, and education. Information sharing, consultation, and treatment planning have been accomplished by face-to-face discussion, phone conversations, meetings, written requests, letters, and sharing of articles and information. As a psychologist, I have needed to obtain information from my pediatric colleagues about specific illness symptoms, medications for particular illnesses, and the course of particular physical conditions. Some of my questions for my pediatric colleagues have included the following: What are the typical symptoms of someone with duodenitis? What medications are used to treat this problem? What is the time frame in which one would expect to see some symptomatic relief?

On the other hand, my physician colleagues have been interested in questions related to diagnostic criteria for such problems as eating disorder or depression, developmental expectations for children, and information concerning the effectiveness of psychological treatments. Such information sharing typically involves discussions regarding patients and is accomplished by face-to-face discussion, telephone conversation, or by the exchange of relevant articles.

Management of Referrals and Communication

Our main contacts involve informal meetings in the office. My office time is shared twice a week with two of the physicians and once a week with the other physician. To initiate a referral, one of the physicians writes an initial letter to me explaining the need for the referral and other pertinent information. He or she will then send additional letters after his further contacts with the patient and family. The other physicians are more likely to use informal face-to-face discussions or telephone calls to make referrals. Initially, before the practice became much busier, our meetings concerning research and clinical care were scheduled regularly. Now they are infrequent. If a patient is to be admitted as an inpatient, and psychological services are requested, I am usually notified ahead of time. If a patient is scheduled to be admitted for specific behavioral treatment as an inpatient, e.g., for a problem such as encopresis, I am always contacted ahead of time, and a multidisciplinary treatment plan is formulated that includes nursing, child-life, and social work.

My working relationships with my physician colleagues have developed over the course of our 9-year association. I am now functioning as an independent professional who is also an integral part of the practice. In this regard, I help to set policy for the practice as a whole concerning such issues as the clinical management of school avoidance in patients with various symptoms, the conduct of parent groups, etc. Such issues are typically discussed at one of the physicians' practice meetings.

Case Examples of Clinical Consultation

Clinical consultation has been a primary vehicle for collaboration in our practice. For example, one common and always difficult referral question has been, "Is there a psychological etiology to the patient's abdominal pain complaint?" One example of the management of such a referral problem was Jamie, a 10-year-old girl with an 8-month history of abdominal pain complaints and more recently school avoidance. Before the onset of her abdominal pain complaints, she had been healthy and attending school without problems. During an initial hospitalization, an extensive series of tests produced no conclusive physical findings. She lived with her mother who had many medical problems including seizures, diabetes, and stomach complaints. Her parents were divorced 5 years ago, but her father lived close by. Presenting as a cheerful, cooperative 10-year-old child, Jamie stated that when she was sick her parents came together to see her. She was in no apparent distress until asked how she was feeling, to which she responded, "My stomach hurts all the time." She denied sad feelings or fears, but when asked if she had any worries, she responded immediately, "My mother." She reported that her mother had been taken by ambulance to the hospital while she had been at school and that she had returned home to an empty house, extremely frightened. She also reported that in the past few months she had been responsible for giving her mother insulin injections. Jamie acknowledged that "my mom has pains in the same places I do." During a second hospitalization, another series of tests was completed, and the results again indicated no significant physical findings.

A meeting with the parents indicated that Jamie's mother had significant anxiety regarding her own physical problems and that she was intently focused on finding a physical cause for Jamie's pain. Jamie's mother felt that her daughter had the same stomach problems she did. However, she saw no connection between her own behavior and her daughter's abdominal pain. My hypotheses about factors that may have influenced Jamie's pain included her attempts to bring the family together, her fears regarding her mother's illness, and her mother's modeling of maladaptive pain behaviors.

A meeting was held with the physicians, the family, and me to discuss the diagnostic findings and to begin the process of helping the family appreciate the relationship of Jamie's pain complaints to other family issues. The medical and psychological information was presented conjointly, along with recommendations for an outpatient treatment plan consisting of close medical monitoring and psychological intervention (including individual and family therapy). The family accepted this recommendation. Jamie eventually experienced a marked reduction in the frequency and intensity of her pain complaints and an increase in her school attendance.

A high level of collaborative treatment is needed to manage children with complex combinations of medical and psychological problems, as shown by the case of Alice, a 14-year-old girl with a 3-year history of severe ulcerative colitis. Her initial clinical course and management were uneventful. However, her illness worsened, and eventually surgery was required. The surgery was accomplished in a three-step process. The first surgery removed the patient's colon and created an ileostomy, and two further surgeries then eliminated the pouch. In addition to dealing with the extraordinary stresses associated with these operations, Alice also had to deal with significant family problems that were heightened as a result of her illness. Individual psychotherapy and family sessions and intermittent conjoint meetings with the physician were necessary to provide sufficient support for her and her family.

The process of consultation in our practice has not been one-sided. For example, I have initiated consultations to my physician colleagues concerning the health status of children such as the following. Bill is a 15-year-old diagnosed with nonspecific colitis that had been under control for the past 2 years with a combination of medications. Psychological treatment was initiated because of a highly stressful family situation, including an actively alcoholic brother, that had been affecting the patient's illness. During the course of his psychological treatment, Bill had a significant flare-up of his colitis and was referred back to his physician to reevaluate his medications and make sure that they were still appropriate.

BENEFITS OF COLLABORATIVE PRACTICE

Facilitating the Engagement of Children and Families in Assessment and Intervention

One significant benefit of this collaborative practice has been the increased recognition by my physician colleagues of the impact of psychological factors on children with GI disorders and the need to address them in a comprehensive management plan. Moreover, the close working relationship among the physicians and me has facilitated patients' and family members' awareness that many GI problems do not reflect a simple dichotomy between "physical" and "psychological" etiologies (see Chapter 6). My introduction to families as a member of the practice has also enhanced their acceptance of the need for psychological assessment and intervention. For example, giving patients and family members an opportunity to meet me informally prior to a scheduled visit has helped to allay some of their fears about seeing a psychologist. Moreover, my physician colleagues save time and energy by dealing with a psychologist whom they trust, who has specialized expertise with GI disorders, and who they know will accept their referrals.

Mutual Learning

Our collaborative practice has also improved the level of interdisciplinary communication necessary to care effectively for children with complex GI disorders and their families (Whitehead & Schuster, 1985). For example, my improved knowledge of the symptoms, medical treatment, and medication side effects of GI disorders has allowed me to make more accurate diagnostic distinctions and treatment recommendations. On the other hand, my physician colleagues have learned the specific criteria for various psychological problems and how to inquire about the presence of family stress and their effects on children's health. Moreover, they have also developed a better appreciation of the contributions and the limits of psychological intervention with their patients. Our modeling and mutual reinforcement of specific behaviors with children and families, e.g., not responding anxiously to certain physical symptoms, setting limits with patients and families on school avoidance, etc. have also improved our collective clinical management.

Problems in Collaborative Work

The main difficulty in this collaboration has involved the intense, fast-paced nature of a busy medical subspecialty practice where immediate clinical issues are the primary concern. Most recently, the demands for clinical psychological services have been increasingly difficult to manage, especially because physicians, psychologists, and nurses outside of our practice have begun to refer patients for psychological service. Given such demands, there often is not enough time to discuss cases consistently and thoroughly on an ongoing basis. We use letters and chart notes as a substitute for more personal interactions around specific patients. However, if a critical issue arises, personal contact can easily be made. Problems in communication, scheduling, or differences in perspective concerning treatment approaches have been solved by discussion.

Not surprisingly, research has been largely overshadowed by the pressing, immediate demands of this clinical practice. When the practice was formed, I received a small grant to conduct and evaluate groups for the families of children with IBD. However, it has not been possible to continue or develop additional research.

Professional isolation is another potential limitation of this model of practice. Psychologist colleagues have not been immediately available for consultation or support. Having the sole responsibility for conducting psychological interventions with a very complicated patient population has also been stressful. My experience suggests that psychologists in such specialty practices should develop a network of psychologist colleagues in their community and stay abreast of new developments in psychological treatments appropriate for chronic illness populations.

INTEGRATING NEW SERVICES INTO THE PRACTICE

One of the distinct benefits of working closely in a multidisciplinary practice such as this is the opportunity to offer a wide range of services to meet patients' and families' needs. During my postdoctoral year with this service, I became increasingly aware of the special emotional demands on parents of children with IBD. Many parents were very interested in discussing their worries about their child's future and long-term prognosis, including their child's ability to have a family or maintain a job. To address such concerns, we formed a parent support group. The first group consisted of 12 parents who met consecutively for 6 weeks and then for three subsequent meetings. The focus of this group was primarily educational but also provided the opportunity for emotional support. One year later, another parent group using the same format was formed on a different side of town. Parents who participated were energized by their initial group experience, and they wanted to continue their positive experience by providing information to other parents. Subsequently, a 1-day educational workshop was planned and implemented by the parents. Speakers included a psychologist, physicians, and nutritionists from the community. In addition, parents from the practice presented a panel discussion of issues relevant to them. This workshop was free and open to the general public. The evaluations from the audience were very positive, and it was also a very energizing experience for the parents who organized it. Further workshops have been held on a biannual basis on topics such as school-related problems, insurance issues, and management of noncompliance.

Videotaping has also been used extensively for patient and family support and education. My physician colleagues have made a video about IBD that discusses epidemiology, nutrition, and recent advances in medication treatment concerning this condition. I also made a videotape discussing typical psychological reactions to having IBD and issues that patients and families have found particularly difficult. In addition to their use with parent groups, these tapes are available to borrow on an outpatient basis or to use when a child is in the hospital. Feedback from patients and families has been very positive.

To address needs that were expressed by other parents, a videotaped interview with a mother of an encopretic child was also made. This mother eloquently described her troubled feelings about her child's problem and her reaction to medical and psychological treatment. Because encopresis is an "embarrassing" problem and one that is not widely discussed, many parents feel alone and isolated in managing it. In this regard, a number of mothers have asked for a support group for parents of encopretic children.

Another related service has been the beginning of a children's library that contains books related to clinical management issues in the practice, e.g., digestion and elimination, toilet training. Children have responded well to the introduction of these books as part of therapeutic intervention.

I have also shared information with other health care professionals by doing lectures and in-service training to nurses concerning psychological factors as they relate to IBD, encopresis, abdominal pain, and other GI problems. Our group has presented at pediatric grand rounds at our hospital. Recently, I was asked by a different teaching hospital in our community to give two lectures on encopresis and abdominal pain to psychiatric residents. As part of my clinical work, I have also visited schools and presented information to teachers and children concerning IBD.

FUTURE IMPLICATIONS

In considering whether to enter a practice like the one described here, potential collaborators need to consider the congruency of professional values, their ability to communicate effectively, the strength of their mutual interests, and their ability to manage administrative issues. Our ability to communicate with one another has been critical to the success of our endeavor. Moreover, our strong mutual interest in pediatric GI problems has also been important to our collaboration.

Administrative and legal issues are very important to consider in a practice of this type (see Chapter 12). Various arrangements are possible. For example, independent psychologist practitioners with a particular interest and expertise in pediatric GI problems could cultivate referrals from pediatric gastroenterologists without joining the practice. However, it may be advantageous to be part of the same practice so that members can join the same insurance plans. In this practice, I joined a number of insurance plans at the same time as my physician colleagues and had no difficulty being accepted.

Finally, it will be important to document how the combined psychological/medical treatment that is offered in this practice results in improved care and outcomes for children with GI problems, as compared with more traditional models. Our service data suggested that children with certain problems such as recurrent abdominal pain were referred more frequently for psychological consultation than in typical practice settings (Edwards, Mullins, Johnson, & Bernardy, 1994). Our impression is that children treated by this multidisciplinary approach received more efficient psychological services sooner and felt better faster than would have been otherwise possible. Research that validates our clinical experiences and hypotheses would have important clinical and fiscal implications.

14

Consultation in an Adolescent Medicine Clinic

SUSAN L. ROSENTHAL

NEED FOR PSYCHOLOGICAL SERVICES IN ADOLESCENT MEDICINE

Adolescent medicine was identified as an area of special interest over 30 years ago, and the Society for Adolescent Medicine, which currently has about 1,200 members, was established in 1968. Adolescent medicine is a growing specialty and has been given subspecialty status in pediatrics. Initial board exams were given in 1994. Many pediatricians view adolescents as having special health care needs, e.g., confidential care around sexuality, mental health issues, and drug and alcohol use, that require additional training (Irwin, 1986). A survey of pediatricians in private practice indicated that 32% did not accept new patients beyond 15 years. Those pediatricians with specialized adolescent medicine training were more likely to have appropriate clinical equipment, to manage sexuality and substance use concerns, and to provide anticipatory guidance in key areas than those without training (Marks, Fisher, & Lasker, 1990).

The need for adolescent medicine physicians to be both comfortable and willing to address the psychosocial needs of their patients (Stiffman, Earls, Robins, & Jung, 1988) and to communicate with adolescents and families concerning sexuality has frequently been described (Klein, 1993; Croft & Asmussen, 1993). Moreover, the major causes of mortality among

SUSAN L. ROSENTHAL, Ph.D. • Division of Adolescent Medicine, Children's Hospital, Pavilion Building, Elland and Bethesda Avenues, Cincinnati, Ohio 45229-2899.

adolescents have shifted from communicable diseases to psychosocial problems. Violent deaths, i.e., homicide, suicide, and accidents, account for the majority of deaths in adolescents. The major morbidities of adolescence include teenage pregnancy, drug and alcohol use and abuse, tobacco use, and sexual and physical abuse of adolescents (Blum, 1987). Also, disabling conditions ranging from chronic illnesses to developmental disabilities are increasing in prevalence, particularly in the adolescent years (Siegel, 1987). All of these data support the need for high-quality psychosocial services within the confines of a primary care adolescent medicine clinic.

Adolescent medicine physicians report a strong orientation toward addressing psychosocial problems (Biro & Rosenthal, 1990). However, physicians' management of the difficult demands of psychosocial assessment and intervention with adolescent patients and their families is not optimal (Marks, Malizio, Hock, Brody, & Fisher, 1983; Smith, Mitchell, McCauley, & Caldeson, 1990; Swedo & Offer, 1991). Moreover, training models to enhance physicians' management of these problems have not been well delineated. Biro and Rosenthal's (1990) survey noted that only 32% of adolescent medicine physicians received what they considered to be "formal mental health" training, and only 53.8% of these felt that their training had been adequate. However, these same physicians reported spending a mean of 20% of their time with patients who, by their definition, had primary mental health problems and 33% of their time with patients who had a mixture of mental health and organic problems.

Unfortunately, little has been written describing how other professionals such as psychologists should participate in the training of adolescent medicine physicians. Moreover, although psychologists can and do provide important services in adolescent medicine clinics, their specific roles have not been well described. To address this need, this chapter describes the role of the psychologist in consulting to and collaborating with physicians within an adolescent clinic and the implications of this work.

CONSULTATION ISSUES IN AN ADOLESCENT CLINIC

Background Information Concerning the Clinic

The experiential information in this chapter is drawn from the author's 5 years of experience in an adolescent clinic that is affiliated with a large pediatric teaching institution in a primary and tertiary care center. This adolescent clinic provides care to a racially and economically mixed neighborhood and subspecialty care to a larger metropolitan area. The patients are of Caucasian (49%) and African-American (50%) descent. Approximately 60% of patients are covered by Aid to Dependent Children and Medicaid, 25% have private insurance carriers, and the remainder have several different payment sources, including self-pay. In a typical year, there are approximately 900 new visits and 5,500 return visits. The clinic has received federal funds from the Maternal and Child Health (MCH) Bureau for over 15 years to provide interdisciplinary training in the field of adolescent health care. Psychiatric consultation was first described in this clinic in 1974 (Seligman & Rauh, 1974). The involvement of psychology prior to the funding of the MCH grant was largely through research projects.

The current director of the clinic is the original director. He has been consistently supportive of psychology's involvement in interdisciplinary clinical care, training, and research. Over time, as expectations within the medical center have changed, he has supported an evolving role of psychology, which has moved from primarily providing clinical care within the clinic to a broader role involving hospital-wide teaching activities and clinical research. There is grant support for the provision of training in five disciplines: medicine, nursing, psychology, social work, and nutrition. Grant funding for a psychologist's salary has ranged from 100% to a current level of 60%. The grant has also funded a stipend for a psychology trainee. In addition, this particular clinic also provides services and training in special education. Traditionally, patients have entered the clinic with referrals to medical/nursing, reproductive health care, psychology/social work, or nutrition services. In this clinic, primary medical care is provided by both physicians and nurse practitioners.

The clinic provides a full range of mental health services. The "psychosocial team" consists of faculty and "trainees" in both social work and psychology. These trainees include graduate students in social work or psychology, predoctoral interns in psychology, and post-master's fellows in social work. One interesting feature of this setting is that referrals for mental health treatment are made to the psychosocial team rather than to a particular discipline. However, specific consultative requests within the clinic are made to social work and psychology faculty depending on availability. Consultative requests from other clinics/divisions or from inpatient services usually are also made directly to psychology. Therapy cases are divided among the psychosocial team. Typical presenting problems include affective or behavioral difficulties, family problems, psychosocial problems associated with chronic illness, and school problems.

There are many issues that pertain to a psychologist's role within an adolescent medicine clinic. In this discussion, these issues will be organized around training, clinical service, and research. Case examples will be used to illustrate relevant issues.

Training

An important and continuing function of a pediatric psychologist is providing training for fellows and continuing supervision/consultation to medical faculty. In 1991, the *Ad Hoc* Fellowship Standards Committee of the Society for Adolescent Medicine identified 11 core knowledge content areas for adolescent medicine physicians, including normal adolescent psychosocial development, health assessment and management to include common acute and chronic medical problems with special emphasis on those conditions that place adolescents at risk, and the diagnosis and management of adolescents with developmental disabilities (*Ad Hoc* Fellowship Standards Committee, SAM, 1991). However, little has been written outlining policies for the most effective ways of training the fellows both in implementing and utilizing mental health services.

Our clinic is part of an academic institution and receives training grant funds from the Bureau of MCH for interdisciplinary training. Seminars and clinical consultation have been the major methods of teaching. Ongoing seminars taught by psychology have included psychological development of adolescents, developmental psychopathology, psychological assessment, and the impact of chronic illness. Examples of special topics taught by psychologists are issues of juvenile sex offenders, identification and treatment of ADHD, and a program to reduce violent behavior in African-American youths. Social workers traditionally have taught the seminars on family development and assessment.

The teaching approach within this clinic relies heavily on the physician fellow or faculty to evaluate his/her own personal and professional strengths and weaknesses accurately in assessing the patient's needs. However, routine cases are not reviewed, so it is difficult to address problems that the physician may be missing entirely. One approach for dealing with this problem is to offer to provide continuing supervision by meeting regularly with the physician. Such supervisory sessions can be organized around a specific topic, e.g., communication skills, or a specific patient. The psychologist can meet with the physician and a particular patient or discuss the patient with the physician before or after the patient is seen.

In our settings, all 1- and 2-year adolescent medicine fellows are evaluated every 6 months by an interdisciplinary team of three faculty members, only one of whom is from the fellow's discipline. Requests for the psychologist's supervision around topical issues have occurred when areas of weakness were identified as a result of this evaluation. Recommendations for supervision have been made for patients who presented with personality and/or behavioral problems that interfered with their medical care. However, the psychologist's offers for supervision typically have not been well utilized by the physicians. Other training difficulties arise because physician fellows may not identify the same weaknesses that faculty members have identified or may not accurately assess their competencies and deficits. Some tensions are also created by the fact that physicians are not accustomed to the same type of supervision utilized in the training of psychologists. Even with the opportunity afforded by close individual supervision, it has been very difficult for physicians to discuss process or relationship issues that arise between them and their patients. On the other hand, highly specific, patient-focused supervision, either in a group or individually, has proven to be a more comfortable format for most physicians.

One important component of training is helping the physician learn to set priorities for clinical management and effectively utilize community resources. Such training opportunities usually arise when the physician presents a multiproblem family for which the request is either for treatment or a nonspecific "Help!" request, such as the following. An adolescent girl who had not attended school for the past several months secondary to "panic attacks" had a history of sexual abuse and lived with a chronically ill mother. In addition, her mother also cared for a preschooler with attention deficit disorder. The physician did not identify a clear consultation question but was overwhelmed and did not know what to do with this family. The consultation focused on helping this physician to determine priorities for intervention, to assess the family's involvement with community services, and to determine the most appropriate services.

Training Psychologists

To address the need to train mental health professionals to provide services to adolescents (Rosenthal & Biro, 1990), we have also had training psychology graduate students provide care to adolescents in a medical setting and consultation to adolescent medicine physicians. In our clinic, advanced clinical psychology graduate students participate in a year-long, 20-hour a week fellowship, which includes experiences in psychotherapy, assessment, and consultation. They attend the adolescent medicine seminars and interact regularly with fellows from other disciplines. We have found that much of the interdisciplinary training in the clinic occurs spontaneously and informally. Psychology interns also participate in the adolescent medicine seminars and carry a small caseload. Because of their limited time in the clinic, they are less well integrated into the program.

One important aspect of training psychologists to work within adolescent medicine settings is to familiarize them with the psychological and health problems of adolescents, e.g., normal pubertal and sexual development, methods for preventing pregnancy or the acquisition of sexually transmitted diseases. Receiving such training early in the course of their graduate training may impact students' career choices. Several students who initially had a clinical rotation within our clinic have gone on to complete dissertations that developed from their clinical work with adolescents on such topics as the relationship between formal operational thought and contraceptive use (Cohen, 1993) and the relationship between parental monitoring and risk taking in adolescents with juvenile rheumatoid arthritis (Nash, 1994). These students have benefited from the conjoint expertise of psychology and medicine faculty within our clinic. Moreover, well-established relationships between faculty members have facilitated data collection. This type of collaborative research training may help address the continuing need to enhance psychological research with adolescent populations (Elkins & Roberts, 1988).

Enhancing Physicians' Knowledge of Adolescent Development

Adolescent medicine physicians often have limited training in developmental issues, particularly regarding the nuances of family relationships during adolescence. Adolescent medicine physicians often focus on the adolescents' striving for independence and needs for confidentiality without understanding such developmental needs in the context of family culture and expectations. The adolescent medicine literature rarely addresses appropriate ways of involving parents in the health care of adolescents while simultaneously addressing the adolescent's need for confidentiality (Rosenthal, Biro, Cohen, Succop, & Stanberry, 1994). An example of this type of referral is an adolescent female who had been receiving her medical care in our clinic and was known to be impulsive. She was diagnosed with cervical dysplasia and was told that she would need a cervical biopsy. Her mother was not with her at the appointment and was not informed that this information had been shared with her daughter. When her daughter became suicidal, the mother was angry that she had not been involved in her daughter's care. In this case, the physician provided standard "confidential care" without considering the individual family relationships and needs. For example, this adolescent's mother was well aware of her daughter's sexual behavior, including her sexual risk taking, so that confidentiality was not a major problem in this case. Although the relationship between mother and daughter was at times volatile, this relationship was generally a positive, stabilizing force for the teenager. Had the physician in this case considered this relationship, he would have recognized the advantages of involving the mother in her child's care.

A related example is a young woman who was placed on birth control pills as part of an effort to induce her menstrual cycle rather than as a method of contraception (this patient was not sexually active and did not believe in having intercourse prior to marriage). The use of birth control pills even for medical reasons turned out to be very upsetting to this Catholic family, including the patient. A family member eventually explained that "no woman in her family had ever used birth control." Fortunately, the family had an excellent relationship with their medical and psychological care providers, and these issues were eventually discussed and resolved.

Clinical Care

Because mental health difficulties often influence the health status of adolescents, an integrated, comprehensive approach to providing services for this population is critical (Takanishi, 1993). Optimal care may require the pediatrician and the psychological consultant to have a strong relationship with each other as well as with the patient (Stabler, 1988). This kind of collaborative approach appears most useful when patients have a "mixture" of mental health and organic difficulties that are very difficult to separate, when patients are having difficulty adjusting to a clearly identifiable organic problem, or when patients exhibit high-risk behaviors with both psychological and health consequences. An example of a patient for whom the psychologist's involvement aided in the provision of comprehensive care is a young woman who presented with polycystic ovary disease, hypertension, depression, and family difficulties. She dropped out of school and had numerous somatic complaints. The psychologist and the physician worked very closely with this young woman. Her medical problems were discussed jointly in order to ensure that the medical information was conveyed in a way she could understand and to alleviate her anxiety regarding her physical symptoms. Eventually, this young woman began to acknowledge that some of her somatic symptoms related to stresses in her life. She began to contact the psychologist when she had functional abdominal pain rather than the physician. As she became less depressed, she used medical services more appropriately.

Adolescent medicine physicians provide not only primary care but subspecialty care as well. Other medical subspecialty services will often refer to the adolescent clinic when concerns regarding adolescents' dangerous risk-taking behaviors are identified. Such referrals are often most appropriately handled either by a psychologist or collaboratively by a physician and a psychologist. For example, one teenager was referred from our rehabilitation service after having injured her leg in a diving accident at a pool. Her history indicated that she was engaging in multiple risk behaviors including unprotected intercourse and alcohol use. The adolescent medicine physician completed a gynecological exam and counseled her regarding safe sex practices. The psychologist helped to establish a school reentry plan and addressed issues of decision making. The care of adolescents with chronic fatigue syndrome also requires a high level of collaboration between psychologists and adolescent medicine physicians as well as with other medical services (Rosenthal, 1993).

Research

Pediatric psychologists can also contribute to the research training and academic productivity of an adolescent medicine clinic through their collaborative efforts. Psychologists who work with adolescent medicine physicians have opportunities to apply their knowledge of psychological measurement and research design to important public health problems (Zaslow & Takanishi, 1993), e.g., sexually transmitted diseases, biological and psychological determinants and implications of sexual intercourse, and acquisition of sexually transmitted disease (Rosenthal, Biro, Succop, Cohen, & Stanberry, 1994).

Although an interdisciplinary approach to the research problems of adolescent health has important advantages, several issues need to be negotiated to make such a collaboration work. It may be up to the psychologist to help his or her colleagues recognize the benefits of the collaborative relationship. Physicians are generally unfamiliar with findings published in the psychological literature and may have difficulties appreciating the subtleties of developmental theory. On the other hand, most psychologists do not understand the fine points of relevant medical information such as pubertal development. Collaborators need to make difficult decisions about the appropriate audiences for presentation and publication of findings (Drotar, 1989).

COLLABORATIVE ISSUES AND PROBLEMS

A recurring theme throughout this chapter has been the tension between the appropriate clinical management of behavioral and psychological morbidities encountered among adolescents and the importance of physicians' accurate evaluation of limits of their own competence to treat such problems. One challenge for the psychologist who works in an adolescent medicine setting is to help physicians accurately evaluate their management skills, learn new skills, and seek appropriate supervision and consultation from other professions. However, this can be a very difficult task because psychologists and adolescent medicine physicians often have very different views on a wide range of professional issues, including management of relations with patients. For example, one physician in our clinic drove a patient home one day and gave her money. This was a patient for whom he had been the primary care provider. The physician did not seek supervision to discuss the implications of his decision, nor did he understand the possible impact of his behavior on his future professional relationship with this patient. This issue only came to light incidentally.

Other common consultation dilemmas arise in helping adolescent medicine physicians to address adolescents' family problems in a balanced manner. Many adolescents who present with psychological difficulties are in the midst of intense struggles with their parents. Adolescents and parents often want the care provider to see the identified problems the way they do and align with their side of the conflict. However, some adolescent medicine physicians are poorly prepared to develop an alliance with both generations and typically are more supportive of the adolescent. In addition, they may not appreciate the need to examine the impact of their own adolescent struggles on their view of their patients' conflicts with their parents.

FUTURE DIRECTIONS

This chapter has provided an initial description of the relationship between adolescent medicine physicians and pediatric psychologists. Some of these experiences may be unique to a clinic that has been funded to provide training for adolescent medicine specialists; others are more generalizable. This chapter has focused predominantly on clinical intervention with adolescents' psychological problems. The opportunity to foster healthy development among nonclinical adolescent populations is another important avenue for pediatric psychologists (Takanishi, 1993). It is my hope that this report will stimulate others to describe the roles of pediatric psychologists in various adolescent medicine settings.

Pediatric psychologists can also play a critical role in providing care to adolescents in community practice settings. In fact, surveys of adolescent medicine physicians indicate that the majority have access to psychologists who function in many capacities ranging from direct service to consultation (Rosenthal & Biro, 1990). However, in order for psychologists to provide quality care to adolescents, they must be trained to evaluate and treat the psychological morbidities of adolescence. Such training should include a thorough understanding of the typical developmental concerns of adolescents, e.g., sexuality, substance use, depression, and an understanding of family development. Evaluation of the efficacy of methods of training and service delivery to adolescent populations is also needed to facilitate collaborative relationships between psychologists and adolescent medicine specialists.

15

Psychological Consultation in Family Medicine

PEGGY CRAWFORD

Psychologists have made substantial inroads in developing collaborative work with pediatricians. However, there are significant opportunities for collaboration with other physician groups that should not be overlooked. For example, psychologists and other professionals, especially social workers, engage in collaborative teaching, practice, and research in academic family practice settings. Campbell, McDaniel, and Seaburn (1992) described several basic premises of family systems medicine that underscore the relevance and importance of behavioral science in this specialty and opportunities for psychologists. These include the primary importance of the biopsychosocial model (Engel, 1977), the emphasis on the family as the most important context in which illness occurs, and the recognition that the practice of family systems medicine requires collaboration between health care providers and mental health professionals. Moreover, the accrediting body of family medicine training mandates the presence of a behavioral science curriculum taught by nonphysician (e.g., psychologist or social work) faculty in family practice training programs. Such curricula include content on assessment and management of psychosocial problems, human development, and doctor–patient relationships (Armstrong, Fischetti, Romano, Vogel, & Zoppi, 1992). Collaborative office practice between family therapists (who may or may not be psychologists) and family practitioners has also been reported (Glenn, Adkins, & Singer,

PEGGY CRAWFORD • Mellon Center for Multiple Sclerosis, Cleveland Clinic Foundation, 9500 Euclid Avenue, Cleveland, Ohio 44195.

1984). The large numbers of children who are seen in family practice settings provide collaborative opportunities for pediatric psychologists that have not been well described. The purpose of this chapter is to describe issues related to psychological consultation in a family practice setting in an academic medical setting.

DESCRIPTION OF SETTING

The Hassler Center for Family Medicine, owned and operated by a 500-bed general community hospital, is the medical office for a family practice residency program. This center is also affiliated with Case Western Reserve University School of Medicine and serves as the training site for 18 residents in family practice. The Center's staff includes six board-certified family physicians, a pediatrician, a pediatric nurse practitioner, a patient education nurse, two part-time psychologists, and a part-time doctor of pharmacy. The Center provides a full range of medical services to adults and children and completes 10,000 patient visits per year.

During their 3-year training program, residents spend increasing amounts of time in the Family Medicine Center seeing patients during office hours. This provides an opportunity to develop a caseload of patients with whom the residents can work on an ongoing basis. During the first year of training, the residents spend one half-day in office hours and the remainder of their time in month-long hospital rotations. By the third year, they spend four half-days seeing patients, with the remainder of their time on electives and covering the family practice inpatient service. Over the course of the residency, they are exposed to psychologists through a number of formal and informal mechanisms, including behavioral science conferences, a required rotation, and working directly with behavioral science faculty on clinical cases.

TYPES OF ACTIVITIES CONDUCTED BY PSYCHOLOGISTS

Psychologists are involved in a variety of clinical and educational activities in this family practice center. Clinical activities include psychological evaluations and interventions for children, adults, and their families. Formal teaching activities include behavioral science conferences held twice a month, focusing on topics related to one of several themes designated for the year, and the month-long behavioral science rotation required of all second-year residents. Many of the clinical activities carried out in conjunction with residents and, less frequently, faculty physicians function as informal training experiences. In addition, one of the psychologists participates in weekly sitdown rounds where all inpatient cases are reviewed and hospital teaching rounds.

Clinical Services and Teaching

Initial psychological assessments of children and adults referred by other faculty and residents are completed by the psychologists in collaboration with a resident or faculty member, if this is requested. Approximately 15–20 referrals are made each month for psychological evaluation. Of these referrals, approximately 60% are children, and 40% are adults. Most of the referrals are made by residents. In approximately half of the cases, residents specifically request that they be involved in at least the initial evaluative portion of the process. For child referrals, the primary presenting problem is most often disruptive and/or oppositional behavior at home and/or at school, sometimes in conjunction with questions about possible attention deficit disorder. Other common presenting problems among children include physical and sexual abuse, adjustment to divorce or death of a parent, depression and anxiety, and recurrent complaints of physical problems without any identifiable organic cause. The primary reason for adult referrals is anxiety and/or depression. Other reasons for adult referrals include adjustment to divorce, marital problems including domestic violence, and emotional distress complicating medical management.

When possible, the initial psychological interview is arranged to accommodate the referring resident's schedule. Although this would seem like a relatively straightforward task, it is often complicated by other resident responsibilities including monthly rotations that take the residents out of the Family Practice Center for significant periods of time. Even when their time can be scheduled, residents are frequently interrupted by phone calls and pages. One component of the educational process for residents is the psychologist's review of the patient's medical record. This process can be instructive for the resident who may have inherited the patient from another resident and had minimal contact with him or her up to this point. As a result of the chart review, it is not unusual to find that some adult patients have been medicated for years for symptoms consistent with anxiety and/or depression with little or no follow-up between requests for medication refills and no referral for mental health services. In addition, many patients have long histories of stress-related physical symptoms with minimal intervention other than medication.

Initially, some residents are more comfortable in the observer role while the psychologist takes primary responsibility for the interview. In doing so, the psychologist provides a role model of how to take a useful psychosocial history. During the interview, pertinent but previously unknown information such as the patient's past use of mental health services, significant life experiences, and a family history of psychological disorders can be elicited. Residents, who are often hesitant to broach potentially emotionally laden or highly charged subjects themselves with their patients, express surprise at how much information patients are willing to share when simply but skillfully asked.

Each of the two part-time psychologists spends approximately one-third of her time providing direct clinical services alone or in conjunction with a resident. Because the center is open two evenings a week and a half-day on Saturday, this increases flexibility and the chances of involving both parents in child cases and both spouses in marital therapy. A few residents continue their participation beyond the initial evaluation phase and become involved in cotherapy sessions. The level of participation varies according to the resident's level of interest and comfort. One resident participated in a series of eight sessions with one of her patients, a 40-year-old married woman who had been blind since infancy as a result of exposure to oxygen as a premature infant. She had experienced chronic anxiety for many years and had been receiving medication, but in recent months her distress has increased, disrupting her sleep and day-to-day functioning in response to interpersonal problems. Although the resident was initially uncomfortable and unclear concerning her role in cotherapy, she gradually became more active in the sessions by asking questions, clarifying issues, and providing feedback to the patient about her behavior and emotional state. By participating in this counseling process, the resident was able to reinforce the woman's behavioral gains and maintain consistent expectations for her at her medical follow-up visits. Over several months, the patient's anxiety level dropped significantly as she developed new coping strategies, and the number of her nighttime emergency calls fell to zero. In addition to modeling how to take a useful psychosocial history, the psychologists' involvement in cotherapy can help residents identify and practice therapeutic interventions that can be used during brief office visits and telephone contacts.

Formal Teaching Activities

The Behavioral Science Rotation. All residents complete a month-long second-year rotation. This concentrated experience exposes the residents to a number of family systems concepts such as thinking of the family as a system organized by interpersonal structures (e.g., boundaries, roles, and coalitions) and processes (e.g., enmeshment, disengagement, and triangulation) that enable it to be both stable and adaptable over time. During this month, the residents participate in didactic sessions on various topics including the application of family systems concepts, use of genograms, identification and assessment of childhood and adult disorders they are likely to encounter in their office practice, and issues related to the management of chronic illness.

One goal of the rotation is to help residents learn to appreciate the family relational context of symptoms and illness, i.e., that symptoms and illness influence and are influenced by the family. This rotation also provides residents with the opportunity to review the clinical or research literature in an area of particular interest and then to present on this topic to the resident and faculty group. One of the most useful clinical experiences during this rotation has been to have the residents and psychologist jointly interview one or more of the patients and families from their own caseload. Often these are patients or families about whom the resident has a hunch that underlying psychological issues and family dynamics may be complicating their adherence to treatment recommendations. The psychologist's involvement in the coassessment of patients from the residents' own caseload, rather than unfamiliar patients, has proved to be very meaningful and useful to the residents, who then have an opportunity to follow up on identified issues as they see their patient for ongoing medical care.

In one such case, a resident had been following a man in his early 30s with serious heart disease who had recently been told that he would need a heart transplant in the coming year. In preparation for the transplant, the patient had been instructed to make several life-style changes including stopping smoking, avoiding stress, and switching to a low-fat diet because he was significantly overweight and had elevated cholesterol. In addition, he had recently stopped working because of fatigue and had been forced to give up his apartment as a result of financial difficulties. The resident was very conscientious and had developed a good relationship with this patient, but now she was feeling very frustrated with the patient because he had not stopped smoking as she had recommended. She viewed this behavior both as detrimental to his present health as well as a possible threat to his receiving a heart transplant.

During the first of two joint interviews with this young man, he articulately described the many losses he had experienced, not just in relation to his recent heart disease but in his life in general. One year prior to the diagnosis of his heart disease, his mother had died of cancer. He had nursed her through this illness and identified her as the one person to whom he felt close and his only real confidant. In addition, one of his older brothers had major heart surgery in recent months, and the young man had not shared the news of his own diagnosis for fear of causing his brother more distress. Concerning his smoking, he acknowledged that although this behavior was not good for him, he continued to smoke as a means of soothing himself when distressed. He also pointed out that he had already given up so much and felt the need to hold onto something. The meaning of this behavior, in the context of multiple losses, was previously unknown to the resident, who had viewed the smoking simply as noncompliant and self-destructive. She had felt puzzled and disappointed about why this man who clearly trusted her as his physician did not change his behavior simply because she had told him to do so.

This case raised a number of important teaching points. First, the meaning of the patient's "noncompliant" behavior was more complex than initially appreciated by both the patient and the resident. With some encouragement the patient was able to describe the meaning of the behavior, thus producing better understanding for both the patient and the resident. As a result, the resident felt less frustrated with the patient and with herself for not having more influence over her patient. Second, the thorough psychosocial history revealed that the patient's current losses were clearly part of a series of losses and helped to place his current experiences in a meaningful context. Third, by identifying the coping strategies that had been typically used by this young man prior to the diagnosis of his heart disease, it became clear that most of them were now unavailable to him (his mother), or he had been counseled to give them up (e.g., eating, working, and smoking). Because he has given up everything else, smoking had a special meaning to him. Finally, this young man pointed out that no matter how much he trusted his physician, his immediate needs to reduce his distress and soothe himself overrode his physician's. During the course of these two interviews, the resident not only found out information about her patient but learned a few things about herself as well. For example, she found to her surprise that it was her patient and not she who was in control of his behavior. After conducting these joint interviews, she felt more comfortable talking with her patient about emotional issues and how they affected his medical care. This facilitated their ongoing work together.

Rounds. Sitdown rounds as well as hospital walk rounds provide regular opportunities for the psychologist to identify psychosocial and family issues that help residents and faculty understand patients' behavioral and emotional responses to illness. Sitdown rounds are held weekly to review all patients hospitalized on the family practice service. The rounds are attended by all third-year residents, the physician faculty advisor for the week, and the psychologist. Notes of pertinent psychosocial information are kept by the psychologist as a means of providing continuity from week to week. This has been particularly helpful in planning care for patients with chronic illnesses who are repeatedly admitted to the hospital. These discussions have revealed that physicians often hesitate to ask about emotional health when the patient's chief complaint concerns physical symptoms or when a physical problem is identified. However, more detailed inquiry about psychological influences has turned out to be particularly important in situations in which patients appear to be making a poor recovery after adequate medical intervention. In such instances, a psychosocial history may reveal important information such as recent negative life events, losses, and/or interpersonal problems that have resulted in increased emotional distress that could be complicating recovery from physical illness. Although many patients are not comfortable about bringing up these issues themselves, they are often relieved to be asked and given an opportunity to discuss their concerns.

One example of such a case is that of a 25-year-old woman who had been admitted to the hospital several days earlier with severe abdominal pain and vomiting. Although the source of her pain was quickly identified and treated, she continued to complain of abdominal pain, took nourishment poorly, thus necessitating the continued use of intravenous fluids, and remained lethargic, spending most of her time sleeping. When this case was reviewed at the sitdown rounds, several residents expressed concern about the inconsistency between her expected and actual response to treatment. When the psychologist inquired about the young woman's psychosocial history and emotional state, the resident in charge of the inpatient service expressed some concern that the woman might be depressed because her affect was flat, and she seemed withdrawn. The resident indicated that she had not been sure how to broach the subject with the patient since she had been admitted for abdominal pain and seemed focused on her physical symptoms. A request was made by the resident that the psychologist interview the woman about possible depression later that same morning during hospital rounds.

In the course of a brief interview, the psychologist asked the woman if there has been any recent changes in her life. Within minutes the woman was in tears talking about the recent breakup of a 5-year relationship with her live-in boyfriend. She went on to describe how depressed she had been over the past month and how this depression had been accompanied by disrupted sleep, weight loss, withdrawal from her friends and usual activities, and poor concentration on her job. When asked if she would consider talking further with one of the psychologists about her concerns, she indicated that she had been in counseling off and on for several months with the other psychologist at the family practice center. Within the hour, the woman was again in contact with her therapist, and therapeutic continuity was preserved. This very brief intervention at the bedside demonstrated how important it is to inquire routinely about psychosocial issues with patients who present with a range of physical symptoms. In spite of this woman's experience with a family practice psychologist and the significant level of her depression, she had not spontaneously offered any of this information during her 5-day hospital stay. However, she quickly revealed a host of emotionally laden issues in response to a few questions.

OBSTACLES TO COLLABORATION

The previously described activities are but a few brief examples of the type of work psychologists can do in a family practice setting. Although they can be rewarding activities, teaching and clinical consultation in a family practice setting are not without significant problems. Collaboration between behavioral scientists and family physicians is affected by differences in training, language, theoretical models, and working style as well as lack of support and professional recognition, and isolation from behavioral science colleagues (McDaniel & Campbell, 1986). In my work, I have noted a discrepancy between the family-centered philosophy of family medicine and the practical problems involved in integrating this philosophy into patient care and teaching. One of the most salient practical problems is that of time. Office visits are often not more than 15 minutes in length, and this limits what can be addressed aside from the chief complaint. In addition, there are frequent disruptions to continuity of patient care related to limited availability of any one physician's office hours. For example, it is not unusual for a patient to see two or three different physicians (usually residents) during the treatment and follow-up of one acute illness episode. This is often as frustrating to the residents as it can be to the patient. Such discontinuity in patient care certainly limits detection of more subtle psychosocial issues that often affect patient compliance.

Another obstacle in collaborating with family physicians is that many of them, including faculty members, are not comfortable addressing psychosocial issues. Consequently, residents may have little reinforcement or role modeling for identifying psychosocial problems and concerns. Even when complex problems such as domestic violence are identified, there is a tendency to approach these situations as if they were acute illnesses rather than the chronic problems they often signify. This often results in simplistic and short-sighted recommendations to try to fix the problem as soon as possible.

In spite of these obstacles, there are many opportunities for psychologists to provide high-quality clinical and teaching services as well as expertise in applied research in family medicine (Campbell *et al.*, 1992). In such settings, the psychologist can increase the physicians' awareness about and comfort with psychosocial issues so that they will inquire about them, understand how they can impact complex health- and illness-related behaviors, and refer patients for psychological services when appropriate. Finally, other opportunities for psychologists in family practice include inpatient consultation and working with patients who have difficulties adjusting to chronic illnesses and adhering with treatment regimens.

16

New Opportunities for Collaboration

Implications

These psychologists' descriptions of their consultation efforts in disparate settings and with various collaborators, including family practitioners, adolescent medicine physicians, pediatric gastroenterologists, and general pediatricians in community practice, illustrate several common themes. These include issues in developing collaborative relationships, the challenges of integrating psychology into medical practice, and managing tensions in collaboration.

DEVELOPING COLLABORATIVE RELATIONSHIPS

Each of these consultants' experiences illustrate various issues in collaborative relationships. For example, Hurley faced the difficult burden of building relationships with pediatricians in a community practice without having prior contact with them. In order to accomplish this difficult task, she had to convince these pediatricians that a psychologist would be a useful addition to their practice. In order to do so she needed to address her future colleagues' questions and concerns, especially whether a psychologist would be responsible for her own referrals. Once Hurley established a collaborative relationship with her pediatric colleagues, she faced other difficult interprofessional issues such as the need to participate in decision making in the practice.

Cunningham's experience provides a contrasting example because her collaborative practice evolved from a prior professional relationship with her pediatric colleagues. During a period of several years, she had an opportunity to work out various collaborative issues, such as communication with her colleagues and decisions related to the practice. These contrasting relationship histories may account for the differences in the psychologist's level of involvement in decision making described in these two practices. However, as Cunningham noted, even a long-standing relationship with medical colleagues is not an antidote to communication problems and difficulties in coordinating efforts in consultation.

Rosenthal's and Crawford's presentations of their work illustrate issues in developing collaborative relationships to enhance the teaching of adolescent medicine specialists and family practitioners. In order to be seen as effective teachers in their respective settings, these psychologists needed to convince their physician colleagues that they had something useful and relevant to teach. Moreover, they needed to conduct this teaching in ways that did not unduly threaten their colleagues. Convincing physicians who have been trained to make their own medical decisions that they have something to learn from someone in another profession, i.e., a psychologist, and that such learning can occur without undue loss of professional control is very difficult. In many settings, effective teaching requires the development of an interprofessional relationship in which physicians can learn to trust that the psychologist is sincerely interested in teaching them (as opposed to controlling or diminishing them in some way). In view of the marked variation in physicians' interests and abilities to participate in such collaborative relationships, limits in the overall effectiveness or "take" of teaching efforts that were noted by both Rosenthal and Crawford are not surprising, albeit frustrating.

CHALLENGES OF INTEGRATING PSYCHOLOGY INTO MEDICAL SETTINGS

Each of these consultants' descriptions of their work illustrate the necessity to shape psychology into a tangible product that is useful to physicians and can be effectively integrated into their practice worlds. In starting her practice, Hurley was called upon to present the advantages of psychology in very concrete terms to pediatric practitioners and subsequently to make good on her promises. Her visibility, availability, and the positive response of parents to her services were all tangible evidence of her commitment and utility. In her collaborative practice setting, Cunningham described several interesting ways in which her work was successfully integrated into the practice such as conjoint meetings with her physician colleagues and families, participation in policy decisions concerning how best to manage difficult clinical cases, and planning new services such as parent groups and educational videotapes.

Rosenthal and Crawford provided examples of how psychology can be translated into concrete, practical terms for the purpose of teaching and service. Using somewhat different methods, these authors based their teaching efforts on clinical problems that were of primary concern to their physician colleagues in their respective settings. The challenge of such teaching is to help physicians appreciate alternative explanations of their patients' clinical problems and new approaches to clinical management that they would not have considered on their own. To accomplish this task, psychologist consultants need to help physicians extend their explanatory models of patient and family problems (Katon & Kleinman, 1981). Rosenthal's and Crawford's case descriptions illustrate how consultants may need to help their physician colleagues accept some very difficult psychological truths, e.g., that human behavior is very difficult to change; that practitioners cannot completely control their patients' destinies (yes it is true!). Because they depart significantly from physicians' training and expectations, such educational messages are not always popular, nor are they necessarily sought after. Consequently, it is especially critical to develop formal structures to facilitate the integration of psychology into clinical care, teaching, or research in medical settings (see Chapters 2–4). In Rosenthal's adolescent medicine setting, a formal training program, case conferences and seminars, and supervision and formal evaluations of physician trainees provided such structures. In Crawford's family practice setting, her participation in hospital rounds and the residents' required behavioral science rotation, which allowed them to participate in conjoint assessment and intervention, were clearly important to her efforts.

"IT'S NEVER EASY": MANAGING COLLABORATIVE TENSIONS

In developing their respective new directions in consultation, all of these authors had to wade through some difficult "trial by fire" experiences. None was immune to interprofessional tensions, which are clearly inherent in the collaborative enterprise (Drotar, 1983). These tensions took different forms in different settings, e.g., being excluded from meetings and decisions concerning the practice (Hurley); problems in communication and professional perspective (Cunningham); concerns about physicians' abilities to treat psychological problems and address adolescents' family problems in a balanced way (Rosenthal); discontinuity of patient care, physicians' discomfort with psychosocial issues, and overreliance on the medical model (Crawford). Each of these consultants also managed the obstacles to interprofessional communication, practice, and teaching that were generated by time constraints. Hurley and Cunningham both mentioned professional isolation as an important issue in collaborative practice. Hurley described some useful strategies to counter this problem.

The obstacles to collaboration described by these psychological consultants are generalizable beyond their individual settings (Drotar, 1993), as are the solutions that were articulated or implied. Certainly, all of these authors' efforts illustrated the need for flexible persistence. Successful consultants must somehow learn to roll with whatever collaborative punches are delivered (see Epilogue). In developing and maintaining their programs, each of these psychologists worked very hard to maintain a reasonable level of communication with their physician colleagues despite time constraints and differences in professional perspectives. The ability to maintain a solid level of communication despite significant interprofessional differences also appears to be a critical ingredient of collaborative program development in academic medical settings (see Chapter 8).

In developing their respective programs, these consultants needed to consider carefully the balance of costs and benefits of their collaboration. Accordingly, they may have asked themselves such questions as: How are the differences that I'm having with my physician colleagues affecting the quality of my work? Can these problems be addressed by communication and mutual problem solving? If not, can I live with them? All of these psychologists accommodated in various ways to the very medical cultures and settings that they also struggled to change. This fine juggling act of the roles of catalyst for change (where this is feasible) and "team player" who accommodates to difficult, unchangeable setting characteristics is a way of life for psychologists in medical environments. Not everyone can do it. Not everyone wants to do it. However, successful psychological consultants somehow find a way.

17

Anticipating the Future of Collaboration

Prospective students often ask me such questions as these: What do I think about the future of pediatric psychology? What will be the job market for psychologists in pediatric settings? What kinds of collaborative activities will be most important? Being a pediatric psychologist and not a professional seer, I am not entirely comfortable with my crystal ball. Nevertheless, it is important to anticipate future professional challenges (Drotar, 1991).

What can psychologists and pediatricians expect for the future of their interprofessional relationship? From the extensive nature of collaborative work described in this book, it seems highly unlikely that these productive professional partnerships will disappear. This should come as especially good news for readers who have managed to make it through this book. Interdisciplinary collaboration has emerged as a basic and highly valued activity for the pediatric psychologists of the 1990s (Drotar *et al.*, 1993a). The most important questions then become the following: What kinds of collaborative efforts stand the best chance of flourishing in the future? What factors will promote or threaten these collaborative efforts? Beyond these pragmatic considerations, what types of interdisciplinary collaboration *should* be promoted to ensure adequate attention not only to professional interests but to the health and psychological needs of children and families. This chapter considers these questions.

PEDIATRIC WORK FORCE TRENDS AND PRACTICE PATTERNS

Collaboration depends on the presence of colleagues. What we can anticipate for the future of the pediatric work force is one issue facing our physician colleagues. In November, 1993, the American Academy of Pediatrics (AAP) Committee on Careers and Opportunities published a description of pediatric work force trends that is certainly relevant to this discussion. Contrary to earlier, more dire predictions about the future of pediatrics, this group concluded that there will be a growing market for this specialty (Brotherton, 1991) based on increased numbers of children enrolled in Medicaid and managed health care plans, the increasing number of health services being provided to adolescents (Martinez & Ryan, 1989), and the need to manage new problems related to AIDS, family violence, substance abuse, etc. Moreover, to the extent that health care reform facilitates access to care for children and facilities and enhances the subsidy for training of primary care specialties, which seems likely, continued growth of pediatrics appears to be assured.

What kinds of activities are modern pediatricians engaged in? According to the AMA (Division of Survey and Data Sources, 1993), the main professional activity of the overwhelming number (90%) of the 44,881 self-designated board- and non-board-certified pediatricians was the provision of patient care in offices and hospital-based settings. There are growing numbers of women and international medical graduates in pediatrics. Moreover, compared with other medical specialties, pediatricians are relatively young; 28% are younger than 35 years, with another 35% between 35 and 44 years (AMA Division Survey and Data Sources, 1993). One conclusion that can be drawn from these work-force trends is that there will certainly be sufficient numbers of pediatricians for collaborative practice opportunities. Although there is no large-scale information concerning the numbers of psychologists collaborating with pediatricians in various practice arrangements, it is safe to say that such opportunities remain underutilitized.

CHALLENGES TO COLLABORATION

These projections of the pediatric work force tell us little about the type of pediatrics that will be practiced in the future, especially how children's behavioral and developmental problems will be managed. Practitioners in private practice or community settings continue to face the troubling problem of keeping their practices financially viable. The pediatrician's role in the assessment and prevention of behavioral and developmental pediatrics will depend on how well such activities will be reimbursed. It is not yet clear how the improved access to pediatric care that should occur under health care reform will translate into reimbursement for behavioral services. This is a critical question because behavioral and developmental pediatricians face special problems obtaining reimbursement, given the nature of their services (SBP Committee on Reimbursement, 1992).

Another important question concerns the fate of pediatric colleagues in academic settings, the majority of whom are subspecialists in a particular organ system. Some specialties, especially emergency medicine, have achieved rapid growth in recent years. (Will we eventually see a next generation of emergency room pediatric psychologists?) On the other hand, pediatric colleagues who specialize in behavior and development have had difficulty competing for reimbursement and recognition (Friedman, 1985). Moreover, pediatricians, including behavioral and developmental pediatricians, in academic medical settings face considerable obstacles in fulfilling expectations for research, practice, and teaching (Ledley & Lovejoy, 1993). Despite these problems, the science of behavioral pediatrics has clearly developed (Green, 1993; Shonkoff, 1993). However, specialty boards remain an important but politically difficult next step.

Training the next generation of behavioral and developmental pediatricians has also proven to be a considerable challenge. The Maternal and Child Health Division of the Bureau of Health Services and Care Delivery Assistance has funded behavioral pediatrics fellowship programs for several years. This initiative is laudable. However, many of these programs have had trouble filling their slots. The reasons are complex but may reflect the difficulties of developing careers in academic medical settings (Ledley & Lovejoy, 1993), reimbursement problems, and the absence of specialty certification (J. H. Kennell, personal communication, April 5, 1994).

Should such trends concern pediatric psychologists? Wouldn't fewer pediatric specialists who are trained to manage children's behavioral and developmental psychologists increase the "need" for pediatric psychologists? To the contrary, my view is that psychologists and many behavioral and developmental pediatricians are allies who share many common interests and professional concerns. Someone needs to recognize the need for psychological services, and pediatricians are clearly the gatekeepers. Unless they are trained to recognize psychosocial problems and the role of psychologists in helping them manage problems, they will not make referrals. Many behavioral and developmental pediatricians have assumed leadership roles for training in the psychological aspects of pediatric care and are strong advocates for these programs (Davidson, 1988). In the absence of pediatric colleagues to support if not champion the need for their skills, some pediatric psychologists may well have difficulty flourishing in academic medical departments (Drotar, 1991) or in pediatric psychology community practice (see Chapters 12 and 13).

Psychologists in academic settings face many of the same problems as their pediatric colleagues in developing resources for their programs and managing difficult work-related demands. In many programs, clinical services have been a primary source of revenues. However, there are several problems with this strategy. Obtaining adequate reimbursement for psychological services has been a continuing problem. As faculty devote more time to services in an effort to meet quotas for revenue, they will inevitably be drawn away from teaching and research activities, limiting academic and teaching productivity and causing frustration (Drotar *et al.*, 1993a). Consequently, diverse strategies to support program development will certainly be needed (see Chapter 8).

IMPACT OF HEALTH CARE REFORM

At the time of the writing of this chapter, marked changes in the entire structure of health care services in the United States, including patterns of reimbursement, are on the horizon with health care reform. The Health Security Act of 1993, the Clinton Administration's proposal for modifying the nation's health care system, would benefit children and their families through increased access for uninsured and underinsured children and their families, which is a problem of national concern (Abraham, 1993). The Health Security Act of 1993 also includes proposals for increasing the number of primary care practitioners through educational reimbursement activities. If these come to pass, the combination of improved access to health care for children and support for pediatricians' professional development would appear to bode well for the pediatric half of the pediatrician–psychologist collaboration.

On the other hand, from a psychologist's standpoint, the Health Security Act has several important limitations (Tomes, 1994). Thus far, psychology has not been listed among the health professions slated to receive federal appropriations for support of students and faculty. In addition, the current mental health benefit, which is the sole source of reimbursement for psychological services, remains limited, especially for children. Finally, as licensed nonphysician providers, psychologists are to be included in health care reform as mental health rather than as primary care providers (Rodgers, 1993). Thus far, the unique preventive services that are offered by pediatric and child health psychologists to children with chronic conditions (Drotar & Bush, 1985) or in primary care, including psychological services that reduce utilization of medical care (Finney *et al.*, 1991), have not been included in the package of mental health benefits. Moreover, there is continuing concern that the Health Securities Act could have a devastating effect on psychological practitioners, including pediatric psychologists, by severely curtailing reimbursement.

At this time, it is not at all clear whether the Clinton plan will be the one that is passed. The headline of the March 1994 edition (Vol. 25, No. 3) of the *APA Monitor* read "Rating the Alternatives to Clinton's Plan." A wide range of proposals, all improving access to health coverage but not necessarily guaranteeing it, and with very different packages for mental health coverage, were described. In this same issue, the titles of various columns reflected the level of professional concern about health care reform, e.g., APA President Ronald Fox: "Health Care Changes Wreak Anxious Times" (p. 3); APA senior policy advisor for Health Care Reform, Bryant Welch: "Mental Health Battles Echo Jurassic Park" (p. 5). In the same issue, an article entitled, "Alliances Are Key to Practitioner Survival" (p. 32) peaked my collaborative interests, so I read on:

> To stay afloat amid the changing health-care market place, psychology practitioners should establish relationships with other professionals, allowing them to share administrative expenses as well as collaborative patient care advise American Psychological Association practice staffers; only through such alliances will psychologists be able to compete in the increasingly integrated and managed marketplace. (Sardella, 1994, p. 32)

Now this sounds a bit like collaborative practice, doesn't it? The above admonition is based on the notion that almost all of the plans for health care reform that are currently being considered involve a managed care model in which solo practitioners and groups or networks compete for contracts with health care plans that serve regional alliances. Some of the potential implications of managed care for collaborative work seem clear. It will be increasingly important for psychologists to develop and sustain professional relationships with primary care, especially those in large groups, because they control access to patients. On the other hand, solo psychology practitioners should have increasing difficulties.

In all likelihood, the cost-containment policies inherent in managed care will also force a reallocation of costs away from hospitalization to primary care. Mental health practitioners will be expected to provide a full range of services at the lowest possible cost. With increased emphasis on documenting quality of care and patient satisfaction, cost-effective methods of evaluation and monitoring of services should become increasingly important to pediatric psychologists (Finney *et al.*, 1991; Kanoy & Schroeder, 1985). Moreover, creative ways of demonstrating the efficacy and cost savings of pediatric psychology services to managed care alliances will most certainly be needed. Otherwise, managed care programs will have no way of identifying the special expertise of pediatric psychology practitioners over more general service providers. Finally, whatever plan for health care reform is finally accepted, the implementation will vary markedly by state. This will intensify the need for psychologists, including pediatric psychologists, to be very active in state-level advocacy concerning health care reform and in documenting the scope and efficiency of psychological services.

In combination with such documentation, the need to disseminate the work of pediatric psychologists to public and elected officials at local, state, and national levels will be critical. Most people are not aware of the kind of services, training, and research that are provided by pediatric psychologists in collaboration with their professional colleagues.

STRATEGIES TO ENHANCE FUTURE COLLABORATIVE EFFORTS

My palm reading of future trends suggests that several strategies will be useful in meeting the future challenges of interdisciplinary collaboration.

Specialization

Although managed care could very well temper this trend, clinical service, teaching, and collaborative work should become increasingly specialized (Drotar, 1991, 1994) (see Chapters 3, 6, and 12–15). Many pediatric subspecialists prefer collaborating with psychologists who share their interest and expertise with a pediatric population.

However, as our activities become increasingly diverse and specialized, we will face the difficult challenge of how best to maintain our identities as psychologists, both in individual settings and in our profession at large (Drotar, 1991). As psychological research activities become increasingly focused on specific pediatric conditions, this will inevitably threaten the development of generalizable knowledge and necessitate new research strategies (Drotar, 1994).

Collaborative Clinical Management

The pediatric psychologists of the future will need to join their pediatric colleagues to develop services for pediatric populations whose needs are not fully addressed within current patterns of care and may not be effectively addressed in health care reform. For example, many children with chronic conditions receive less than optimal psychological services (Sabbeth & Stein, 1990). Some of these problems, e.g., recurrent somatic symptoms, have considerable costs for the health care system (Finney *et al.*, 1991). Effective delivery of mental health services to economically disadvantaged children is another important challenge (Tarnowski, 1991) that will undoubtedly require a high level of collaboration among pediatricians, psychologists, and other professions.

Collaborative Training Activities

Cooperative training activities will continue to be important to develop the pediatrician and psychologist collaborators of the future (Davidson, 1988). As noted by the AAP Committee on Psychosocial Aspects of Child and Family Health (1993), in order to manage the problems of the "new morbidity," pediatricians will need to expand their knowledge base concerning risk factors, normal variations, behaviors affecting children's physical health, e.g., medical noncompliance, as well as skill development, e.g., interviewing skills, detection of behavioral and developmental problems, referral skills, and management. The increasingly strenuous agenda for training future pediatricians to manage psychological disorders in their practices would appear to provide important opportunities for psychologists. As health care professionals whose clinical skills are especially relevant to pediatric practice, psychologists are in an excellent position to help train pediatricians. However, to fulfill this role, psychologists will need to be trained in consultation and collaboration (see Chapter 11).

Collaborative Research Opportunities

I can envision continued expansion of opportunities for collaborative research with pediatricians. Leaders of behavioral and developmental pediatrics have consistently underscored the importance of collaborative interdisciplinary research for the development of this field (Green, 1993; Shonkoff, 1993). Research opportunities abound in charting psychological outcomes and developing interventions for emerging high-risk pediatric populations. The psychological outcomes and risk factors for a whole host of new populations, e.g., HIV infection, cocaine exposure, and for more familiar problems, e.g., child abuse and neglect, have not been well documented. Moreover, the field would certainly benefit from research concerning the efficacy of interventions for important but difficult clinical problems, e.g., chronic illness, recurrent pain.

To develop the knowledge base concerning interdisciplinary collaboration and consultation, research concerning the efficacy of psychological services, including multidisciplinary studies (see Chapters 6 and 10), must be done. Collaborative research concerning factors that enhance pediatric identification and prevention of behavioral and developmental problems will be particularly important. Pediatric psychologists can look to the work of the first two winners of the research contribution awards from the Society of Pediatric Psychology (SPP), John Spinetta and Lizette Peterson, for models of researchers who have enhanced scientific knowledge of problems that are of practical interest to pediatric colleagues. For example, Spinetta extended knowledge of the psychological adaptation of children with cancer and underscored the importance of professional communication with such children (Spinetta & Maloney, 1978). Peterson's research has illuminated our understanding of interventions that are designed to reduce children's distress in response to surgery and painful medical procedures (Peterson, Ridley-Johnson, Tracy, & Mullins, 1984) and more recently concerning childhood injury (Peterson, Harbeck, & Moreno, 1993). The combination of methodological rigor and clinical relevance that has characterized such work will never become obsolete.

COLLABORATION BETWEEN AAP AND APA

One very important direction for the future will be to expand the level of collaboration among pediatricians and psychologists through their major professional organizations, AAP and APA (Wright, 1985). Each of these organizations has a complex, profession-specific agenda. Nevertheless, certain areas of mutual professional interest, e.g., diagnosis and coding of children's behavioral problems and public policy, have been a focus of collaboration that should continue in the future.

Task Force on Coding for Mental Health in Children

One primary obstacle to collaborative clinical care among pediatricians and psychologists has been the absence of a common diagnostic language to describe the full range of behavioral problems and environmental situations that are encountered in practice. The *DSM-III* (and now *-IV*) categories cover only a small range of problems that are seen by pediatricians in practice. Most pediatricians do not utilize the *DSM* in their practices, nor do they conceptualize clinical problems in accord with this system. Moreover, many psychologists are also uncomfortable with the lack of a health and empirical foundation for the *DSM*.

Based on agreement among several primary care specialties that the *DSM-IV* would not provide a suitable, adequate coding system for primary care even with substantial revision, the Task Force on Coding for Mental Health in Children was developed under the leadership of Mark

Wolraich, a pediatrician at Vanderbilt University. The American Academy of Pediatrics along with several other professional groups has strongly supported this task force by contributing financial and program staff support. The Task Force has the following mandate: (1) to develop a classification schema that is compatible with the *DSM-IV* but addresses the broad range of symptoms and problems that are seen in the primary care setting and thus has clinical utility for pediatrics (as well as clinical psychology); (2) encompasses a wide spectrum of problems, not just disorders; (3) as much as possible is based on research; and (4) has a developmental focus.

To tackle this considerable agenda, the Task Force has been structured around interdisciplinary work groups, each of which includes pediatricians, child psychiatrists, and at least two psychologists, many of whom are quite recognizable as prominent pediatric or clinical child psychologists. The titles of the work groups reflect the wide range of behavioral and developmental problems and stressful situations seen in pediatric practice: (1) Environmental and Interactional Factors, (2) Response to Physical Conditions, (3) Emotions and Moods, (4) Disruptive Behaviors, (5) Somatic Psychic Interface, (6) Cognitive Perceptual Problems, and (7) Severity and Functional Assessment. Each of these groups has been charged to develop definitions for problems in the domain and algorithms for diagnosis that can be used by practitioners in primary care.

These efforts should benefit pediatricians, psychologists, and family practitioners who conduct their practice in primary care. Although these efforts were not planned with the explicit purpose of reimbursement, they could have such implications. An expanded coding system would also have the important advantage of giving practitioners and researchers a more accurate vocabulary for diagnosis and management and for research with subthreshold clinical problems (including health-related problems) that are nowhere to be found in the *DSM-III-R* and will not be included in the *DSM-IV*. This effort has also been a focal point for APA (through Division 12, Section 1, SPP, and Section 5, Clinical Child Psychology) to collaborate with AAP on an issue of mutual professional interest. The current timetable is to develop a first working draft of the system that will be available for critique and feasibility testing by pediatricians, psychologists, and other groups in the summer of 1994. Field trials will then be conducted to collect data to support and modify the coding system.

Collaborative Advocacy in Service Development and Policy

In all likelihood, psychologists and pediatricians and their colleagues will contend with an ever-increasing array of clinical problems that reflect the influence of poverty and limited access to health care (Baumeister, Kupstas, & Woodley-Zanthos, 1993; Haggerty, 1989; Wise & Meyers, 1988). These problems will challenge us to reach far beyond the scope of available resources and models of service delivery. For example, in a slice of professional life from some of my recent clinical consultations, I was asked to assess a 4-year-old child who was admitted to the hospital for treatment of smoke inhalation in a fire and who had possible neurological and developmental problems related to this event. She was one of three children in her family who had been hurt. I also saw a 2-year-old admitted for developmental assessment in connection with severe lead poisoning, her third such admission in 1 year. A third consultation concerned an adolescent who was admitted because he attempted to hang himself; he reported that he and his brothers were playing "911." Pediatricians and psychologists in hospitals throughout the country face similar and even worse scenarios. When such problems come cascading one after another, they can not only erode one's sense of efficacy but shatter any remaining illusions that the fabric of our society is really intact.

There are clearly no ready solutions to the widespread problems that seriously threaten the physical and psychological health of children and their families. However, we know that they will not be solved by health care reform. On the contrary, they will require continuing efforts among pediatricians, psychologists, and many other professionals and families to build coalitions that advocate for the needs of children and their families in order to promote more effective services and preventive care for children and families on local, state, and national levels.

Ideally, this agenda should expand existing collaborations between AAP and APA concerning promotion of national policy to enhance the health and well-being of children and their families. The public policy office of APA (B. Wilcox, personal communication, Mar. 28, 1994) noted several important areas of ongoing interorganizational collaboration concerning policy. These are summarized below.

The Impact of Children's Television. To secure passage of the Children's Television Act of 1990, APA organized a small coalition, and AAP was the key additional member. Following enactment of the law, APA and AAP filed a joint "petition for reconsideration" with the Federal Communication Commission (FCC) regarding the rules implementing the act. Specifically, the petition challenged the FCC's claims regarding children's "limited cognitive abilities and attention spans" and the application of this claim to programming requirements.

These organizations have also worked jointly on the TV violence issue. As early as 1986, they began working together in support of legislation to provide the television industry with an antitrust exemption allowing them to meet jointly to discuss means of addressing the problem. More recently, APA started a collaboration through the Public Interest Directorate to stimulate a joint public information campaign on the issue of media violence.

Child Maltreatment. As members of the National Child Abuse Coalition, APA and AAP have worked together for many years on child maltreatment policy issues, especially to secure increased funding for child abuse research, prevention, and service programs. For example, they have collaborated on the reauthorizations of the Child Abuse Prevention and Treatment Act. This has involved working with key Congressional committees in drafting provisions for the legislation.

Child Mental Health. Both the APA and AAP are members of the National Consortium for Child and Adolescent Mental Health Services, an organization representing 23 professional and consumer organizations interested in child mental health. Representatives of these organizations have testified before Congress on funding for child mental health services and training and have lobbied Congress. Finally, AAP and APA have coordinated their efforts on many other policy issues, e.g., lobbying for research funding at the National Institute of Child Health and Human Development (NICHD).

FACILITATING PROGRAM AND PROFESSIONAL DEVELOPMENT

The field of pediatric psychology needs to promote the professional development, satisfaction, and career development of the next generation of pediatric psychologists. To accomplish this task, pediatric psychologists will need to develop and disseminate effective strategies supporting the professional development of teachers, researchers, clinicians, and administrators in this field. This will involve sustained communication of strategies and approaches at professional meetings, through the SPP newsletter, through personal contact, and in journal articles.

My discussions with leaders of pediatric psychology programs and observations of current trends, including projections based on health care reform, suggest that the prospect of securing resources to support the activities of pediatric psychologists in academic medical settings will be increasingly difficult. The most successful programs will be those that have the most comprehensive and effective collaboration with pediatric colleagues. One can also anticipate that entrepreneurial pediatric psychologists will continue to build practices with pediatric colleagues in community settings. We certainly need to keep our colleagues abreast of new collaborative opportunities. I very much hope that this book serves as a catalyst for information exchange in the service of promoting interdisciplinary collaboration in its many forms.

Epilogue

Reflections on Lessons Learned in Collaboration

The experience of writing this book has given me ample opportunity to reflect on the lessons learned from collaborative work. Although these particular lessons draw heavily on one person's experience and should be considered in that light, they may have some generalizability. For this reason, I submit them to you in this epilogue.

WHAT CAN PSYCHOLOGISTS LEARN FROM PEDIATRICIANS?

Collaboration is sometimes portrayed as a unidimensional activity in which psychologists bring their expertise in clinical work, teaching, and research to pediatric colleagues. However, opportunity to learn from pediatric colleagues is one of the most rewarding features of collaboration. Pediatric colleagues have much to offer psychologists and other professionals in their clinical experience and perspective, advocacy efforts, and interest in practical applications of research.

Clinical Experience and Perspective

Most pediatricians have a broad-based knowledge of differential diagnosis and biological determinants of behavior that is equally critical for psychologists (Olness & Libby, 1987). Many pediatric subspecialists have also amassed a wealth of clinical experience in managing the problems presented by children and adolescents with chronic conditions, including the unique experience of caring for such children who are now adults. Another strength of pediatricians stems from their experience with a wide range of children with essentially normal physical and psychological development. Levine (1991) described developmental–behavioral pediatricians as fundamentally longitudinal and developmental in their views and as having a commitment to normality and to normal stylistic variation (as opposed to deviation).

In contrast to clinical psychologists whose contacts with children and families focus primarily on clinical problems, the continuity and longevity of the pediatrician's relationship with parents and children are hallmarks of pediatric practice. These experiences provide a unique opportunity to distinguish normal variations and transitory disturbances from more serious problems. Pediatricians also have opportunities to provide support to families and children who are undergoing significant life stressors.

Advocacy

Many pediatricians are staunch advocates on behalf of children and families at local and national levels. As chair of the Social Concerns Committee of the Society of Behavioral Pediatrics for several years, I had contact with pediatric colleagues who were engaged in advocacy at many different levels, e.g., in testifying before and lobbying Congress, in working with state and local advocacy groups, in international relief efforts, and helping parents advocate on behalf of individual children. Such activities provide important opportunities to form coalitions to enhance public policy to benefit children and their families (see Chapter 17).

Enhancing the Practical Application of Psychological Research

Many pediatricians consistently ask two interrelated questions concerning psychological research: (1) What is the value of this research to pediatric practice? (2) How can it directly benefit my patients? Well-designed research that enhances scientific knowledge does not always have to have an immediate, pragmatic value. However, our pediatric colleagues constantly remind us that psychological research should ultimately have clinically significance.

WHAT MAKES AN EFFECTIVE PSYCHOLOGICAL CONSULTANT?

Another set of lessons learned concerns the attributes of an effective psychological consultant. In my view, the effective consultant is a heroic blend of training and personal attributes.

Training and Experience

To be most effective, psychologists cannot simply transfer traditional training in clinical psychology to pediatric (or other medical) settings. They need to understand the special characteristics of pediatric populations, be familiar with assessment and interventions with specialized clinical problems, and be knowledgeable about setting characteristics and influences. Because each pediatric setting has a unique history of collaboration and faculty and program attributes, experience in several pediatric settings is a helpful perspective builder.

Personal Attributes

Beyond training and experience, I believe that several personal attributes make for a good psychological consultant. These include respect and tolerance for pediatric colleagues, a strong personal and professional identity, pragmatic orientation, professional commitment, and the ability to manage the inherent stresses and changes of medical settings.

An appreciation of one's pediatric colleagues, especially their professional contributions and strengths, can go a long way toward sustaining effective collaboration. Such appreciation should go hand in hand with a healthy tolerance for colleagues' personal foibles, the limitations of medical training, and the impact of setting demands on their interpersonal and interprofessional behavior.

Effective psychological consultation requires a balance between accommodation to the needs of pediatricians and strong professional interests and identity. I believe that professional and personal interests should not be submerged by accommodation. For this reason, one needs to have (or develop) sufficient confidence to advocate strongly for one's point of view concerning patient care, research, etc., and relevant professional issues (see Chapter 6).

From a pediatrician's vantage point, I would think that the most important ingredients in an effective consultant are a strong action orientation and the ability to translate psychological knowledge into a usable form. A successful consultant needs consistently to deliver an extraordinary product: a practical intervention plan that also addresses the complexity of a clinical problem.

One of the most powerful ingredients in my personal recipe for a successful psychological consultant is a high level of professional commitment. Consultants need to document their work and follow through with communications with children, parents, and pediatricians, even when it is not convenient to do so. Moreover, the best consultants will often go beyond minimum expectations by providing additional advocacy and contacts with outside agencies.

SUSTAINING CONSULTATION AND COLLABORATION OVER TIME

Many psychologists who consult pediatric settings find that the conscientious management of their responsibilities is more than a full-time job. Moreover, to sustain a high level of professional performance at the saintly levels that I have described may well be an impossible job, especially because of the stresses to which consultants are exposed. Successful experiences with pediatric colleagues are often counterbalanced by run-ins with physicians who ask the impossible and are just as impossible to deal with. Psychological consultants also have to deal with the stresses of the human condition, with children and adolescents undergoing painful procedures, children who are dying, and women who have been battered and whose children are abused. The high level of stresses that are encountered in pediatric settings requires consultants to develop strong supports to manage these stresses or risk burnout.

In the presence of such stresses, one central question becomes: What strategies can best sustain psychological consultants' energies and professional zeal over the course of time? In my own work, I have found strategies such as setting realistic expectations, developing diverse activities, and renegotiating responsibilities to be helpful.

Setting Realistic Expectations

Psychological consultants need to evaluate whether the many expectations that they and/or others place on them are realistic. Consultants are often in the middle of many competing expectations. For example, a pediatrician wants the child's behavioral problems to be cured; a parent wants his child out of the hospital; nursing staff want the child to take his or her medication, etc. All hope that the consultant can help them. Even the best and brightest of psychological consultants will not be able to please all the relevant parties all of the time. For this reason, psychological consultants need to be realistic about what they can and cannot accomplish. Because of the demands of pediatric settings, it is important to negotiate manageable workloads and reasonable allocation of various responsibilities. Wherever possible, verbal agreements concerning job responsibilities should be put in writing. Although it is not possible to foresee all contingencies, especially in new positions, a written agreement provides guidelines that will make it easier to explain and justify activities both to yourself and to your pediatric colleagues.

Diversity of Activities

In my experience, a diverse set of activities can serve as an antidote to the stresses that are associated with clinical consultation. For example, activities such as teaching and research do not involve patient care and hence provide some distance from high-intensity clinical activities. Diversity and balance in clinical activities may also help to maintain enthusiasm and limit stress.

Flexibility in Managing Change

Psychologists in medical settings experience significant changes in settings, collaborators, department chairs, patient populations, and in their own interests and professional priorities. Consequently, the ability to manage change and renegotiate responsibilities is vital to maintain a sense of efficacy in one's work.

The ability to reallocate my responsibilities to follow my interests has been particularly important to me. As the first full-time psychologist in a large pediatric teaching hospital, Rainbow Babies & Children's Hospital, I developed a clinical consultation service in the first phase of my work, lasting for about 7 years. Gradually, my activities have shifted from a primary emphasis on clinical work to a much greater focus on research.

As I finish this epilogue, I am pondering the next set of my collaborative activities. Along with my pediatric colleagues, I need to complete the data analysis for our study of the cognitive development of Ugandan infants. A pediatric neurologist just contacted me about my observations and thoughts concerning medication management for a child with attention deficit disorder with learning difficulties and a chronic low-level depression. A consultation request concerning a child who is failing to thrive just came in. On the training front, I need to plan a meeting with pediatric pulmonary colleagues to discuss a student's dissertation research project. Yes, still collaborating after all these years.

References

Abraham, L. K. (1993). *Momma Might Be Better off Dead. The Failure of Health Care in Urban America*. Chicago: University of Chicago Press.

Abt, F. (Ed.). (1965). *Abt–Garrison History of Pediatrics*. Philadelphia: W. B. Saunders.

Achenbach, T. M. (1991). *Manual for the Child Behavior Checklist*. Burlington, VT: University of Vermont.

Ack, M. (1974). The psychological environment of a children's hospital. *Pediatric Psychology, 2*, 3–5.

Ad Hoc Fellowship Standards Committee, Society for Adolescent Medicine. (1991). Unpublished document, Joseph L. Rauh, MD, Division of Adolescent Medicine, Children's Hospital Medical Center, 3333 Burnet Avenue, Cincinnati, OH 45229.

American Academy of Pediatrics. (1993a, February). *Status Report on Academy Initiatives*. Elk Grove, IL: Author.

American Academy of Pediatrics. (1993b, November). Pediatric work force statement. *Pediatrics, 92*, 725–730.

American Academy of Pediatrics Committee on Psychosocial Aspects of Child and Family Health. (1993). The pediatrician and the "new morbidity." *Pediatrics, 92*, 731–733.

American Medical Association Division of Survey and Data Sources. (1993). *Physician Characteristics and Distribution in the U.S.* Washington, DC: AMA.

American Psychological Association. (1992). Ethical principles of psychologists and code of conduct. *American Psychologist, 47*, 1597–1611.

Anderson, J. E. (1930). Pediatric and child psychology. *Journal of the American Medical Association, 95*, 1015–1018.

Anderson, J. E. (1956). Child development: An historical perspective. *Child Development, 27*, 181–196.

Armstrong, P., Fischetti, L. R., Romano, S. D., Vogel, M. S., & Zoppi, K. (1992). Position paper on the role of behavioral science faculty in family medicine. *Family Systems Medicine, 10*, 257–264.

Artiss, K. L., & Levine, A. S. (1973). Doctor–patient relation in severe illness. A seminar for oncology fellows. *New England Journal of Medicine, 288*, 1210–1214.

Bailey, D., & Garralda, M. E. (1989). Referral to child psychiatry: Parent and doctor motives and expectations. *Journal of Child Psychology and Psychiatry, 30*, 449–458.

Baker-Ward, L., Gordon, B. N., Ornstein, P. A., Larus, D. M., & Clubb, P. A. (1993). Young children's long-term retention of a pediatric examination. *Child Development, 64*, 1519–1533.

Barkley, R. A., Barclay, A., Conners, C. K., Gadow, K., Gittelman, R., Sprague, R., & Swanson, T. (1990). Task force report: The appropriate role of clinical child psychologists in prescribing of psychoactive medication. *Journal of Clinical Child Psychology, 19* (Suppl.), 1–38.

Baumeister, A. A., Kupstas, F. D., & Wooley-Zanthes, P. (1993). *The New Morbidity: Recommendation for Action and an Updated Guide to State Planning for Prevention of Mental Retardation and Related Disabilities Associated with Socioeconomic Conditions.* Washington, DC: U.S. Department of Health and Human Services, President's Committee on Mental Retardation.

Becker, M. J. (Ed.). (1974). *The Health Belief Model and Personal-Health Behavior.* New York: Slack.

Belar, C. D. (1991). Professionalism in medical settings. In J. J. Sweet, R. H. Rozensky, & S. M. Tovian (Eds.), *Handbook of Clinical Psychology in Medical Settings* (pp. 81–94). New York: Plenum Press.

Bergman, A. B., Dassel, S. W., & Wedgewood, R. J. (1966). Time–motion study of practicing pediatricians. *Pediatrics, 38,* 254–263.

Bergman, A. S., & Fritz, G. V. (1985). Pediatricians and mental health professionals: Patterns of collaboration and utilization. *American Journal of Diseases of Children, 139,* 155–159.

Berkoff, K., & Drotar, D. (1994). Coping styles and health-related behaviors in pediatric and internal medicine house. The role of personality styles, gender, and year of training. *Journal of Developmental and Behavioral Pediatrics, 15,* 162–169.

Berkoff, K., & Rusin, W. (1991). Pediatric house staff's psychological response to call duty. *Journal of Developmental and Behavioral Pediatrics, 12,* 6–10.

Biro, F. M., & Rosenthal, S. L. (1990, March). *Mental health training and perceived competence by adolescent medicine providers.* Poster presented at the Society for Adolescent Medicine Annual Meeting, Atlanta, GA.

Black, M., Dubowitz, H. Hutcheson, J., Berenson-Howard, J., & Starr, P. H. (1994). *Home intervention among children with nonorganic failure to thrive. Results of a randomized clinical trial.* Unpublished manuscript, University of Baltimore, Baltimore, MD.

Blum, R. (1987). Contemporary threats to adolescent health in the United States. *Journal of American Medical Association, 257,* 3390–3395.

Botinelli, C. B. (1975). Establishment of an outpatient psychology screening clinic: Preliminary considerations. *Pediatric Psychology, 3,* 10–11.

Brenneman, J. (1932). Pediatric psychology and the child guidance movement. *Journal of Pediatrics, 2,* 1–16.

Brotherton, S. E. (1991). Career plans of new pediatricians: Results from a survey of residency program directors. *Pediatrics, 88,* 861–866.

Bull, B. A., & Drotar, D. (1991). Coping with cancer in remission: Stressors and strategies reported by children and adolescents. *Journal of Pediatric Psychology, 16,* 767–782.

Burman, K. D. (1982). Hanging from the masthead. Reflections on authorship. *Annals of Internal Medicine, 97,* 602–605.

Campbell, T. L., McDaniel, S. H., & Seaburn, S. B. (1992). Family systems medicine: New opportunities for psychologists. In T. J. Akamatsu, M. P. Stephens, S. E. Hobfoll, & J. H. Crowther (Eds.), *Family Health Psychology* (pp. 193–215). Washington, DC: Hemisphere.

Caplan, G. (1970). *Theory and Practice of Mental Health Consultation.* New York: Basic Books.

Caplan, G., & Caplan, R. B. (1993). *Mental Health Consultation and Collaboration.* San Francisco: Jossey Bass.

Chamberlin, R. W. (1982). Prevention of behavioral problems in young children. *Pediatric Clinics of North America, 29,* 239–248.

Charlop, M. H., Parrish, J. M., Fenton, L. R., & Cataldo, M. J. (1987). Evaluation of hospital-based pediatric psychology services. *Journal of Pediatric Psychology, 12,* 485–503.

Christophersen, E. R. (1982). Incorporating behavioral pediatrics into primary care. *Pediatric Clinics of North America, 29,* 261–296.

Christophersen, E. R. (1983). Behavioral analysis of well-baby and well-child care. In M. L. Wolraich & D. K. Routh (Eds.), *Advances in Developmental and Behavioral Pediatrics* (Vol. 4, pp. 109–123). Greenwich, CT: JAI Press.

Christophersen, E. R. (1991). Toileting problems in children. *Pediatric Annals, 20,* 240–244.

Christophersen, E. R. (1992). Discipline. *Pediatric Clinics of North America, 39,* 395–411.

Christophersen, E. R. (1993). *Pediatric Compliance: A Guide for the Primary Care Physician.* New York: Plenum Press.

Christophersen, E. R., & Abernathy, J. (1982). Research in ambulatory pediatrics. In D. C. Russo & J. W. Varni (Eds.), *Behavioral Pediatrics: Research and Practice* (pp. 299–332). New York: Plenum Press.

Christophersen, E. R., & Gyulay, J. E. (1981). Parental compliance with care seat usage: A positive approach with long-term follow-up. *Journal of Pediatric Psychology, 6,* 301–312.

Christophersen, E. R. & Long, N. (1987, May). Pediatric inpatient consultations. *Newsletter of the Society of Pediatric Psychology, 11,* 3–17.

Christophersen, E. R., Soslan-Edelman, D., & LeClaire, S. (1985). Evaluation of two comprehensive infant car seat loaner programs with 1-year follow-up. *Pediatrics, 76,* 36–42.

Cohen, S. S. (1993). *The relationship between cognitive development and sexual behaviors among college females.* Unpublished doctoral dissertation, University of Cincinnati, Cincinnati, OH.

Copeland, L., Wolraich, M., Lindgren, S., Milich, R., & Woolson, R. (1987). Pediatricians' reported practices in the assessment and treatment of attention deficit disorder. *Journal of Developmental and Behavioral Pediatrics, 8,* 191–197.

Costello, E. J. (1986). Primary care pediatrics and child psychopathology: A review of diagnostic, treatment, and referral practices. *Pediatrics, 85,* 711–716.

Croft, C. A., & Asmussen, L. (1993). A developmental approach to sexuality education: Implications for medical practice. *Journal of Adolescent Health, 14,* 109–114.

Cushna, B. (1968). Psychology and pediatrics. *American Psychologist, 23,* 288.

Daeschner, C. W., & Cerreto, M. C. (1985). Training physicians to care for chronically ill children. In N. Hobbs & J. M. Perrin (Eds.), *Issues in the Care of Children with Chronic Illness* (pp. 458–477). San Francisco: Jossey-Bass.

Dana, R. H., & May, T. W. (1986). Health care megatrends and health psychology. *Professional Psychology, 17,* 251–253.

Davidson, C. V. (1988). Training the pediatric psychologist and the developmental–behavioral pediatrician. In D. K. Routh (Ed.), *Handbook of Pediatric Psychology* (pp. 507–537). New York: Guilford Press.

Delameter, A. M., Bubb, J., Davis, S. G., Smith, J. A., Schmidt, L., White, N. H., & Santiago, J. V. (1990). Randomized prospective study of self-management training with newly diagnosed diabetic children. *Diabetes Care, 13,* 492–498.

Dobos, A. E., Dworkin, P. H., & Bernstein, B. A. (1994). Pediatricians' approaches to developmental problems: Has the gap been narrowed? *Journal of Developmental and Behavioral Pediatrics, 15,* 34–38.

Drotar, D. (1975). The role of the psychologist in a treatment program for end-stage renal failure. *Pediatric Psychology, 3,* 10–14.

Drotar, D. (1976). Psychological consultation in the pediatric hospital. *Professional Psychology, 9,* 77–83.

Drotar, D. (1977a). Clinical psychological practice in the pediatric hospital. *Professional Psychology, 8,* 72–80.

Drotar, D. (1977b). Family-oriented intervention with the dying adolescent. *Journal of Pediatric Psychology, 2,* 68–71.

Drotar, D. (1978). Training psychologists to consult with pediatricians: Problems and prospects. *Journal of Clinical Child Psychology, 7*, 57–61.

Drotar, D. (1983). Transacting with physicians: Fact and fiction. *Journal of Pediatric Psychology, 8*, 117–127.

Drotar, D. (1985). The role of psychology in behavioral pediatrics. *Journal of Developmental and Behavioral Pediatrics, 6*, 207–208.

Drotar, D. (1988). Failure to thrive. In D. K. Routh (Ed.), *Handbook of Pediatric Psychology* (pp. 71–107). New York: Guilford Press.

Drotar, D. (1989). Psychological research in pediatric settings: Lessons from the field. *Journal of Pediatric Psychology, 14*, 63–74.

Drotar, D. (1991). Coming of age: Critical issues in the future development of pediatric psychology. *Journal of Pediatric Psychology, 16*, 1–14.

Drotar, D. (1993). Influences on collaborative activities among psychologists and physicians: Implications for practice, research, and training. *Journal of Pediatric Psychology, 18*, 159–172.

Drotar, D. (1994). Psychological research with pediatric conditions. If we specialize, can we generalize? *Journal of Pediatric Psychology.*

Drotar, D., & Bush, M. (1985). Mental health issues and services. In N. Hobbs & J. M. Perrin (Eds.), *Issues in the Care of Children with Chronic Illness* (pp. 232–265). San Francisco: Jossey Bass.

Drotar, D., & Ganofsky, M. A. (1976). Mental health intervention with children and adolescents with end-stage renal failure. *International Journal of Psychiatry in Medicine, 7*, 181–194.

Drotar, D., & Ievers, C. (1994). Preliminary report: Age differences in parent-child responsibilities for management of cystic fibrosis and insulin-dependent diabetes mellitus. *Journal of Developmental and Behavioral Pediatrics, 15*, 367–374.

Drotar, D., & Malone, C. A. (1982). The developmental case conference as a method of teaching pediatricians about child development on an inpatient service. *Clinical Pediatrics, 19*, 261–262.

Drotar, D., & Sturm, L. (1988). The role of parent–practitioner communication in the management of nonorganic failure to thrive. *Family Systems Medicine, 6*, 42–53.

Drotar, D. & Sturm, L. (in press). Interdisciplinary collaboration in the practice of mental retardation. In J. W. Jacobsen & J. A. Mulick (Eds.), *Manual of Diagnosis and Professional Practice in Mental Retardation*. Washington, DC: American Psychological Association.

Drotar, D., Ganofsky, M. A., & Makker, S. (1979). Psychosocial intervention in childhood renal failure. *Dialysis and Transplantation, 8*, 73–77.

Drotar, D., Benjamin, P., Chwast, R., Litt, C., & Vajner, P. (1982). The role of the psychologist in pediatric outpatient and inpatient settings. In J. M. Tuma (Ed.), *Handbook for the Practice of Pediatric Psychology* (pp. 228–250). New York: John Wiley & Sons.

Drotar, D., Crawford, P., & Ganofsky, M. A. (1984). Prevention with chronically ill children. In M. C. Roberts & L. Peterson (Eds.), *Prevention of Problems in Childhood: Psychological Research and Applications* (pp. 232–265). New York· John Wiley & Sons.

Drotar, D., Peterson, N., & Berkoff, K. (1992, April). *Cross-cultural research in pediatric psychology. Issues in studying the psychological consequences of HIV infection in Ugandan infants.* Presented at biannual meeting of North Coast Society of Pediatric Psychology, Buffalo, NY.

Drotar, D., Sturm, L., Eckerle, D., & White, S. (1993a). Pediatric psychologists' perceptions of their work settings. *Journal of Pediatric Psychology, 18*, 237–248.

Drotar, D., Fagan, J. F., Olness, K., Hom, D., Wiznitzer, M., Marum, L., Scheurman, M. M., & Ndugwa, C. (1993b, April). *Developmental outcome of Ugandan infants with perinatally acquired HIV infection*. Presented at the biennial meeting of the Florida Conference on Child Health Psychology, Gainesville, FL.

Duff, R. S., Rowe, D. S., & Anderson, F. P. (1972). Patient care and student learning in a pediatric clinical. *Pediatrics, 50*, 839–846.

Edwards, M. C., Mullins, L. L., Johnson, J., & Bernardy, N. (1994). Survey of pediatricians' management practices for recurrent abdominal pain. *Journal of Pediatric Psychology, 19*, 241–254.

Elkins, P. O., & Roberts, M. C. (1988). *Journal of Pediatric Psychology*: A content analysis of articles over its first ten years. *Journal of Pediatric Psychology, 13*, 575–594.

Engel, G. L. (1977). The need for a new medical model: A challenge for biomedicine. *Science, 196*, 126–129.

Enright, M. F., Resnick, R. J., Ludwigsen, K. R., & Deleon, P. L. (1993). Hospital practice: Psychology's call to action. *Professional Psychology: Research and Practice, 24*, 135–141.

Evers-Szostak, M., Schroeder, C. S., & McClure, S. Y. (1991, April). *Pediatric psychologists in private pediatric practices*. Paper presented at the Florida Conference on Child Health Psychology. Gainesville, FL.

Feightner, J. W., & Cadman, D. C. (1992). Preschool developmental screening in primary care of children. In M. Wolraich & D. K. Routh (Eds.), *Advances in Developmental and Behavioral Pediatrics* (Vol. 10, pp. 1–16). Philadelphia: Jessica Kingsley.

Fernberger, S. W. (1932). The American Psychological Association: A historical summary, 1892–1930. *Psychological Bulletin, 29*, 1–89.

Fife, C. A. (1934). The child's family advisor. *Transactions of the American Pediatric Society, 46*, 19.

Finney, J. W., Friman, P. C., Rapoff, M. A., & Christophersen, E. R. (1986). Improving compliance with antibiotic regimens for otitis media: Randomized clinical trial in a pediatric clinic. *American Journal of Disease of Children, 139*, 89–95.

Finney, J. W., Lemanek, K. L., Cataldo, M. F., Katz, H. P., & Fuqua, R. W. (1989). Pediatric psychology in primary health care: Brief target therapy for recurrent abdominal pain. *Behavioral Therapy, 29*, 283–291.

Finney, J. W., Brophy, C. J., Friman, C. J., Golden, A. S., Richman, G. S., & Ross, A. F. (1990). Promoting parent–provider interaction during young children's health supervision visits. *Journal of Applied Behavioral Analysis, 23*, 207–213.

Finney, J. W., Riley, A. W., & Cataldo, M. F. (1991). Psychology in primary care. Effects of brief target therapy on children's medical care utilization. *Journal of Pediatric Psychology, 16*, 447–462.

Fischer, H. D., & Engeln, R. G. (1972). How goes the marriage? *Professional Psychology, 3*, 73–79.

Fox, R. (1957). Training for uncertainty. In R. K. Merten, G. Reader, & P. C. Kendall (Eds.), *The Student Physician* (pp. 123–167). Cambridge: Harvard University Press.

Frank, D. A., & Drotar, D. (1994). Failure to thrive. In R.-M. Reece (Ed.), *Child Abuse. Medical Diagnosis and Management* (pp. 298–325). Philadelphia: Lea & Febiger.

Freidson, E. (1970). *Profession of Medicine: A Study of the Sociology of Applied Knowledge*. New York: Harper & Row.

Friedman, S. B. (1985). Behavioral pediatrics. Interactions with other disciplines. *Journal of Developmental and Behavioral Pediatrics, 6*, 202–207.

Friman, P. C., Finney, J. W., Rapoff, M. A., & Christophersen, E. R. (1985). Improving pediatric appointment keeping with reminders and reduced response requirements. *Journal of Applied Behavioral Analysis, 18*, 315–321.

Geist, R. (1977). Consultation on a pediatric surgical ward. Creating an empathic climate on a surgical ward. *American Journal of Orthopsychiatry, 47*, 432–444.

Gesell, A. (1919). The field of clinical psychology as an applied science: A symposium. *Journal of Applied Psychology, 3,* 81–84.

Gesell, A. (1926). Normal growth as a public health concept. *Transactions of the American Child Health Association, 3,* 48.

Gillman, J. B. (1994). Inflammatory bowel diseases: Psychological issues. In R. A. Olson, L. L. Mullins, J. B. Gillman, & J. M. Chaney (Eds.), *The Sourcebook of Pediatric Psychology* (pp. 135–144). Needham Heights, MA: Allyn & Bacon.

Glenn, M. L., Adkins, L., & Singer, G. (1984). Integrating a family therapist into a family medical practice. *Family Systems Medicine, 2,* 137–145.

Good, M. J., & Good, B. J. (1989). Disabling practitioners: Hazards of learning to be a doctor in American medical education. *American Journal of Orthopsychiatry, 59,* 303–309.

Goodgame, R. W. (1990). AIDS in Uganda: Clinical and social features. *New England Journal of Medicine, 323,* 383–389.

Goodman, J. F., & Cecil, H. S. (1987). Referral practices and attitudes of pediatricians toward young mentally retarded children. *Journal of Behavioral and Developmental Pediatrics, 8,* 97–105.

Gordon, B. N., Schroeder, C. S., & Abrams, J. M. (1990a). Age and social class differences in children's knowledge of sexuality. *Journal of Clinical Child Psychology, 19,* 33–43.

Gordon, B. N., Schroeder, C. S., & Abrams, J. M. (1990b). Children's knowledge of sexuality: A comparison of sexually abused and nonabused children. *American Journal of Orthopsychiatry, 60,* 250–257.

Gortmaker, S. C., & Sappenfield, W. (1984). Chronic childhood disorders: Prevalence and impact. *Pediatric Clinics of North America, 31,* 3–18.

Gram, A. M. (1992). Peer relationships among clinicians as an alternative to mentor–protege relationship in hospital settings. *Professional Psychology: Research and Practice, 23,* 416–447.

Green, M. (1985). The role of the pediatrician in the delivery of behavioral services. *Journal of Developmental and Behavioral Pediatrics, 6,* 190–193.

Green, M. (1993). Behavioral pediatrics: Its past and future. *Journal of Developmental and Behavioral Pediatrics, 14,* 405–408.

Green, M., Boyce, W. J., Finney, J. W., Phillips, S., & Zuckerman, B. S. (1992). The future of behavioral pediatrics research. Moving right along. *Pediatrics, 90,* 830–834.

Grose, N. P., & Goodrich, J. J. (1985). Chronicity and the physician. *Family Systems Medicine, 3,* 190–196.

Gross, A. M., & Drabman, R. S. (Eds.). (1990). *Handbook of Behavioral Pediatrics.* New York: Plenum Press.

Haggerty, R. J. (1982). Behavioral pediatrics: Can it be taught? Can it be practiced? *Pediatric Clinics of North America, 29,* 391–398.

Haggerty, R. J. (1986). The changing nature of pediatrics. In N. A. Krasnegor, J. D. Arasteh, & M. F. Calaldo (Eds.), *Child Health Behavior: A Behavioral Pediatrics Perspective* (pp. 9–16). New York: Wiley & Sons.

Haggerty, R. J., Roghmann, K., & Pless, I. B. (1975). *Child Health and the Community.* New York: John Wiley & Sons.

Halpern, S. (1988). *American Pediatrics: The Social Dynamics of Professionalism: 1880–1980.* Berkeley: University of California Press.

Hamlett, K. W., & Stabler, B. (in press). The developmental progress of pediatric psychology consultation. In M. C. Roberts (Ed.), *Handbook of Pediatric Psychology,* 2nd ed. New York: Guilford Press.

Harvey, B. (1993). New series of essays on pediatric history. *Pediatrics, 92,* 467–468.

Hekelman, F. P., Gilchrist, V., Glover, P., Olness, K., & Zyzanski, S. J. (in press). An educational intervention to increase faculty productivity. *Family Medicine.*

Hoffman, Y. (1992). *Effects of a supportive intervention during labor and delivery on post-partum psychological adaptation of first-time mothers.* Unpublished Ph. D. dissertation, Case Western Reserve University, Cleveland, OH.

Horwitz, S. M., Leaf, P. J., Leventhal, M. M., Forsyth, B., & Speechley, K. N. (1992). Identification and management of psychosocial and developmental problems in community-based primary care pediatric practices. *Pediatrics, 89,* 480–485.

Hughes, J. G. (1993). Conception and creation of the American Academy of Pediatrics. *Pediatrics, 92,* 469–470.

Hurley, K. K., McIntire, D., & Evers-Szostak, M. (1994, April). *Patient perceptions of pediatric psychology in primary care.* Paper presented at the Gulfcoast Regional Society of Pediatric Psychology Conference. New Orleans, LA.

Huszti, H. C., & Walker, C. E. (1991). Critical issues in consultation and liaison. In J. J. Sweet, R. H. Rozensky, & S. J. Tovian (Eds.), *Handbook of Clinical Psychology in Medical Settings* (pp. 165–185). New York: Plenum Press.

Ievers, C., Drotar, D., Dahms, W. T., Doershuk, C. F. & Stern, R. C. (1994). Maternal child-rearing behavior in three groups: cystic fibrosis (CF), insulin dependent diabetes mellitus (IDDM), and healthy children. *Journal of Pediatric Psychology, 19,* 681–688.

International Committee of Medical Journal Editors. (1985). Guidelines on authorship. *British Medical Journal, 2,* 291–292.

Irwin, C. E. (1986). Why adolescent medicine? *Journal of Adolescent Health Care, 7,* 2–12.

Iwata, S., Riordan, M. M., Wohl, M. K., & Finney, J. W. (1982). Pediatric feeding disorders: Behavioral analysis and treatment. In P. J. Accardo (Ed.), *Failure to Thrive in Infancy and Early Childhood: A Multidisciplinary Team Approach* (pp. 197–235). Baltimore: University Park Press.

Johnson, S. B., Silverstein, J., Rosenbloom, J. A., Carter, R. & Cunningham, W. (1986). Assessing daily management in childhood diabetes. *Health Psychology, 5,* 545–564.

Joint Commission on Accreditation of Health Care Organizations (1991). *Accreditation Manual for Hospitals.* Chicago: Author.

Kagan, J. (1965). The new marriage: Pediatrics and psychology. *American Journal of Diseases of Childhood, 110,* 272–278.

Kanoy, K. W., & Schroeder, C. S. (1985). Suggestions to parents about common behavior problems in a pediatric primary care office: Five years of follow-up. *Journal of Pediatric Psychology, 10,* 15–30.

Kanthor, H., Pless, I. B., Satterwhite, B., & Myers, G. (1974). Areas of responsibility in the health care of multiply handicapped children. *Pediatrics, 54,* 779–786.

Katon, W., & Kleinman, A. (1981). Doctor–patient negotiation and other social science strategies in patient care. In L. Eisenberg & A. Kleinman (Eds.), *Relevance of Social Science for Medicine* (pp. 253–279). Boston: Reidel.

Katz, J. (1984). *The Silent World of Doctor and Patient.* New York: Free Press.

Kazak, A. (1989). Families of chronically ill children: A systems and social ecological model of adaptation and challenge. *Journal of Consulting and Clinical Psychology, 57,* 25–30.

Kazak, A. (1993). Psychological research in pediatric oncology. *Journal of Pediatric Psychology, 18,* 313–318.

Kazak, A., & Beele, D. (1993). *Overview of Psychosocial Services, The Children's Hospital of Philadelphia, Division of Oncology.* Unpublished program description, The Children's Hospital of Philadelphia, Division of Oncology, Philadelphia, PA.

Kazak, A., & Meadows, A. (1989). Families of young adolescents who have survived cancer: Social emotional adjustment, adaptability, and social support. *Journal of Pediatric Psychology, 14,* 175–191.

Kazak, A., & Nachman, G. (1991). Family research on childhood chronic illness: Pediatric oncology as an example. *Journal of Family Psychology, 4,* 462–483.

Kazak, A., Stuber, M., Gorchinsky, M., Houskamp, B., Christakis, D., & Fasiraj, J. (1992, August). *Post-traumatic stress in childhood cancer survivors and their parents.* Poster presented at the annual meeting of the American Psychological Association, Washington, D.C.

Kazak, A., Blackall, G., Boyer, B., Brophy, P., Daller, R., & Himelstein, B. (1994a). *Promoting change in pediatric oncology services: A systems oriented pharmacologic–psychologic intervention for procedural pain.* Unpublished manuscript, University of Pennsylvania School of Medicine. Philadelphia, PA.

Kazak, A., Boyer, B., Brophy, P., Johnson, K., Scher, C., Covelman, K., & Scott, S. (1994b). *Procedure-related distress and family adaptation in childhood leukemia.* Unpublished manuscript, University of Pennsylvania, School of Medicine, Philadelphia, PA.

Kennell, J. H., Klaus, M., McGrath, S., Robertson, S., & Hinkley, C. (1991). Continuous emotional support during labor in a U.S. hospital: A randomized controlled trial. *Journal of the American Medical Association, 265,* 2197–2201.

Kirsner, J. B., & Shorter, R. G. (1982). Recent developments in "nonspecific" inflammatory bowel disease. *New England Journal of Medicine, 366,* 775–785.

Klein, S. D. (1993). The challenge of communicating with parents. *Journal of Developmental and Behavioral Pediatrics, 14,* 184–191.

Klerman, L. V. (1985). Interprofessional issues in delivering services to chronically ill children and their families. In N. Hobbs & J. M. & Perrin (Eds.), *Issues in the Care of Children with Chronic Illness* (pp. 420–440). San Francisco: Jossey Bass.

Koocher, G. P. (1980). Pediatric cancer: Psychological problems and the high costs of helping. *Journal of Clinical Child Psychology, 9,* 2–5.

Koocher, G. P., Sourkes, B. M., & Keane, W. M. (1979). Pediatric oncology consultation: A generalizable model for medical settings. *Professional Psychology, 10,* 467–474.

Kucia, C., Drotar, D., Doershuk, C. F., Stern, R. C., Boat, T. F., & Matthews, L. (1979). Home observation of family interaction and childhood adjustment to cystic fibrosis. *Journal of Pediatric Psychology, 4,* 479–489.

LaGreca, A. M., Stone, W. L., Drotar, D., & Maddux, J. E. (1988). Training in pediatric psychology Survey results and recommendations. *Journal of Pediatric Psychology, 13,* 121–139.

Ledley, F. D., & Lovejoy, F. H. (1993). Factors influencing the interests, career paths, and research activities of graduates from academic pediatric residency programs. *Pediatrics, 92,* 611–617.

Levine, M. D. (1990). Presidential address to Society for Behavioral Pediatrics. *Journal of Developmental and Behavioral Pediatrics, 12,* 1–3.

Levine, S. Z. (1950). Pediatric education at the crossroads. *American Journal of Diseases of Children, 100,* 651.

Liese, B. S. (1986). Physicians' perceptions of the role of psychology in medicine. *Professional Psychology: Research and Practice, 117,* 226–277.

Lozoff, B., Jimenez, E., & Wolf, A. W. (1991). Long-term developmental outcome of infants with iron deficiency. *New England Journal of Medicine, 325,* 587–694.

Magrab, P. R. (Ed.). (1978a). *Psychological Management of Pediatric Problems, Vol. 1: Early Life Conditions and Chronic Diseases.* Baltimore: University Park Press.

Magrab, P. R. (Ed.). (1978b). *Psychological Management of Pediatric Problems, Vol. 2: Sensorineural Conditions and Social Concerns.* Baltimore: University Park Press.

Marks, A., Malizio, J., Hock, J., Brody, R., & Fisher, M. M. (1983). Assessment of health needs and willingness to utilize health care resources of adolescents in a suburban population. *Journal of Pediatrics, 102,* 456–460.

Marks, A., Fisher, M., & Lasker, S. (1990). Adolescent medicine in pediatric practice. *Journal of Adolescent Health Care, 11,* 149–153.

Martinez, G. A., & Ryan, A. S. (1989). Pediatric marketplace. *American Journal of Diseases of Children, 142,* 924–928.

Matarazzo, J. D., & Daniel, R. S. (1957). Psychologists in medical schools. *Neuropsychiatry, 4,* 93–107.

McGrath, P. A. (1990). *Pain in Children*: New York: Guilford Press.

Mechanic, D. (1978). *Medical Sociology*. New York: Free Press.

Mensh, I. N. (1953). Psychology in medical education. *American Psychologist, 8,* 53–85.

Mesibov, G. B. (1984). Evolution of pediatric psychology: Historical roots to future trends. *Journal of Pediatric Psychology, 2,* 15–17.

Mesibov, G. B., Schroeder, C. S., & Wesson, L. (1977). Parental concerns about their children. *Journal of Pediatric Psychology, 2,* 15–17.

Meyer, J. D., Fink, C. M., & Carey, P. F. (1988). Medical views of psychological consultation. *Professional Psychology: Research and Practice, 19,* 356–358.

Moise, J., Drotar, D., Doershuk, C. F., & Stern, R. C. (1987). Correlates of psychosocial adjustment among young adults with cystic fibrosis. *Journal of Developmental and Behavioral Pediatrics, 8,* 141–148.

Mullins, L. D., Gillman, J., & Harbeck, C. (1992). Multiple-level interventions in pediatric psychology settings: A behavioral systems perspective. In A. M. LaGreca, L. J. Siegel, J. L. Wallander, & C. E. Walker (Eds.), *Stress and Coping in Child Health* (pp. 371–399). New York: Guilford Press.

Nash, A. A. (1994). *The relationship between monitoring and substance use in adolescents with juvenile rheumatoid arthritis*. Doctoral dissertation, University of Cincinnati, Cincinnati, OH.

Olness, K., & Torjesen, H. (1991). State of the world's children. Developmental-behavioral disorders in a global context. In M. I. Gottlieb (Ed.), *Developmental Behavioral Disorders* (pp. 3–16). New York: Plenum Press.

Olson, R. A., Holden, E. W., Friedman, A., Faust, J., Kenning, M., & Mason, P. J. (1988). Psychological consultation in a children's hospital: An evaluation of services. *Journal of Pediatric Psychology, 13,* 479–492.

Olson, R. A., Holden, E. W., Friedman, A., Faust, J., Kenning, M., & Mason, P. J. (1989). Psychological consultation in a children's hospital. An evaluation of services. *Journal of Pediatric Psychology, 13,* 479–482.

Olson, R. A., Mullins, L. L., Gillman, J. B., & Chaney, J. M. (Eds.) (1994). *The Sourcebook of Pediatric Psychology*. Needham Heights, MA: Allyn & Bacon.

Ottinger, D. K., & Roberts, M. C. (1980). A university-based predoctoral practicum in pediatric psychology. *Professional Psychology, 11,* 707–713.

Perrin, J. M. (1992). Abuse related to new technologies for the health care of children. In M. Wolraich & D. K. Routh (Eds.), *Advances in Behavioral and Developmental Pediatrics* (Vol. 10, pp. 181–194). Philadelphia: Jessica Kingsley.

Peterson, L., & Harbeck, C. (1988). *The Pediatric Psychologist. Issues in Professional Development and Practice*. Champaign, IL: Research Press.

Peterson, L., Ridley-Johnson, R., Tracy, K., & Mullins, L. L. (1984). Developing cost-effective presurgical preparation: A comparative analysis. *Journal of Pediatric Psychology, 9,* 274–296.

Peterson, L., Harbeck, C., & Moreno, A. (1993). Measures of children's injuries: Self-reported versus maternal reported events with temporally proximal versus delayed reporting. *Journal of Pediatric Psychology, 18,* 133–147.

Peterson, N. J. (1994). *The impact of maternal HIV infection on infant-to-mother attachment*. Unpublished Ph. D. dissertation, Case Western Reserve University, Cleveland, OH.

Phipps, S., & Drotar, D. (1990). Determinants of parenting stress in home apnea monitoring. *Journal of Pediatric Psychology, 15,* 385–389.

Pruitt, S. D., McGowan, R. J., Elliot, R. H., Koerner, K., & Mullins, L. (1988, August). *Physician referral patterns as impediments to collaboration in behavioral medicine*. Poster presented at annual meeting of American Psychological Association.

Rae, W. D., & Fournier, C. J. (1986). Ethical issues in pediatric research: Preserving psychological care in scientific inquiry. *Children's Health Care, 14*, 242–248.

Rapoff, M. A., & Christophersen, E. R. (1982). Improving compliance in pediatric practice. *Pediatric Clinics of North America, 29*, 339–358.

Report of U.S. Preventive Service Task Force. (1989). *A Guide to Clinical Preventive Services: An Assessment of the Effectiveness of 169 Interventions*. Baltimore: Williams & Wilkins.

Richmond, J. B. (1967). Child development: A basic science for pediatrics. *Pediatrics, 39*, 645–647.

Roberts, M. C. (1986). *Pediatric Psychology: Psychological Interventions and Strategies for Pediatric Problems*. New York: Pergamon Press.

Roberts, M. C. (1992). Vale dictum: An editor's view of the field of pediatric psychology and its journal. *Journal of Pediatric Psychology, 17*, 785–805.

Roberts, M. C., & Wright, L. (1982). Role of the pediatric psychologist as consultant to pediatrician. In J. M. Tuma (Ed.), *Handbook for the Practice of Pediatric Psychology* (pp. 251–289). New York: John Wiley & Sons.

Rodgers, D. A. (1993, November). Psychology in a vacuum in Clinton plan. *National Psychologist, 2*, 18.

Rogers, J. C., & Holloway, R. L. (1993). Professional intimacy: Somewhere between collegiality and personal intimacy. *Family Systems Medicine, 11*, 263–270.

Rosenthal, S. L., Biro, F. M., Cohen, S. S., Succop, P. A., & Stanberry, L. R. (1994). *Parents, peers, and the acquisition of an STD: Developmental changes in girls*. Unpublished manuscript, University of Cincinnati, School of Medicine, Cincinnati, OH.

Rosenthal, S. L., Biro, F. M., Succop, P. A., Cohen, S. S., & Stanberry, L. R. (1994). Age of first intercourse and risk of STD. *Adolescent and Pediatric Gynecology, 7*, 210–214.

Routh, D. K. (1969). Graduate training in pediatric psychology: The Iowa program. *Pediatric Psychology, 1*, 4–5.

Routh, D. K. (1970). Psychological training in medical school departments of pediatrics: A survey. *Professional Psychology, 1*, 469–472.

Routh, D. K. (1972). Graduate training in medical school departments of pediatrics: A second look. *American Psychologist, 27*, 587–589.

Routh, D. K. (1975). The short history of pediatric psychology. *Journal of Clinical Child Psychology, 4*, 6–8.

Routh, D. K. (Ed.). (1988). *Handbook of Pediatric Psychology*, New York: Guilford Press.

Routh, D. K. (1990). Psychology and pediatrics. The future of the relationship. In A. M. Gross & R. S. Drabman (Eds.), *Handbook of Clinical Behavioral Pediatrics* (pp. 403–414). New York: Plenum Press.

Routh, D. K. (1994). *Clinical Psychology since 1917: Science, Practice, and Organization*. New York: Plenum Press.

Routh, D. K., Schroeder, C. S., & Koocher, G. P. (1983). Psychology and primary health care for children. *American Psychologist, 38*, 95–98.

Routh, D. K., Ernst, A. R., & Harper, D. C. (1988). Recurrent abdominal pain in children and somatization disorder. In D. K. Routh (Ed.), *Handbook of Pediatric Psychology* (pp. 492–504). New York: Guilford Press.

Russo, D. C., & Varni, J. W. (Eds.). (1982). *Behavioral Pediatrics: Research and Practice*. New York: Plenum Press.

Sabbeth, B., & Stein, R. E. K. (1990). Mental health referral: A weak link in the comprehensive care of children and chronic physical illness. *Journal of Developmental and Behavioral Pediatrics, 11*, 73–78.

Salk, L. (1970). Psychologist in a pediatric setting. *Professional Psychology, 1,* 395–396.

Sarason, S. B. (1972). *The Creation of Settings and the Problem of Change.* Boston: Allyn & Bacon.

Sarason, S. B. (1981). *Psychology Misdirected.* New York: Free Press.

Sardella, S. (1994, March). Alliances are key to practitioner survival. *APA Monitor, 25*(3), 32.

Schowalter, J. E., Ferholt, J. B., & Mann, N. M. (1973). The adolescent patient's decision to die. *Pediatrics, 51,* 97–103.

Schroeder, C. S. (1979). Psychologists in a private pediatric practice. *Journal of Pediatric Psychology, 4,* 5–18.

Schroeder, C. S. (1993, August). *Mental health services in outpatient pediatric primary care.* Presented at Annual Meeting of American Psychological Association, Toronto, Canada.

Schroeder, C. S., & Mann, J. (1991). A model for clinical child practice. In Schroeder, C. S., & Gordon, B. N. (Eds.), *Assessment and Treatment of Childhood Problems: A Clinician's Guide* (pp. 375–398). New York: Guilford Press.

Schroeder, C. S., Goolsby, E.,& Stangler, S. (1974). Interdisciplinary training in preventive services in a private, *Pediatric Psychology, 2,* 6.

Schroeder, C. S., Goolsby, E., & Stangler, S. (1975). Preventive services in a private pediatric practice. *Journal of Clinical Child Psychology, 4,* 32–33.

Schroeder, C. S., Gordon, B. N., Kanoy, K., & Routh, D. K. (1983). Managing children's behavior problems in pediatric practice. In M. Wolraich & D. K. Routh (Eds.), *Advances in Developmental and Behavioral Pediatrics* (Vol. 4, pp. 25–86). New York: JAI Press.

Seagull, E. (1979). Writing the report of the psychological assessment of a child. *Journal of Clinical Child Psychology, 8,* 39–42.

Seligman, R., & Rauh, J. L. (1974). Psychiatric consultation in a medical setting for adolescents. *Clinical Pediatrics, 13,* 117–120.

Senn, M. J. E. (1975). Insights on the child development movement in the United States. *Monographs of the Society for Research in Child Development. 40* (nos. 3–4), Serial No. 161, 1–107.

Shonkoff, J. P. (1993). Reflections on an emerging academic discipline: The prolonged gestation of developmental and behavioral pediatrics. *Journal of Developmental and Behavioral Pediatrics, 14,* 409–412.

Siegel, D. M. (1987). Adolescents with chronic illness. *Journal of American Medical Association, 257,* 3396–3399.

Simonian, S. J., Tarnowski, K. J., Stancin, T., Friman, P. C., & Atkins, M. S. (1991). Disadvantaged children and families in pediatric primary care settings: Screening for behavior disturbances. *Journal of Clinical Child Psychology, 20,* 360–371.

Singer, L. T., & Drotar, D. (1989). Psychological practice in a pediatric rehabilitation hospital. *Journal of Pediatric Psychology, 14,* 479–489.

Singer, L. T., & Fagan, J. F. (1984). Cognitive development in the failure to thrive infant: A three-year longitudinal study. *Journal of Pediatric Psychology, 9,* 363–383.

Smith, E. E., Rome, L. P., & Freedheim, D. K. (1967). The clinical psychologist in the pediatric office. *Journal of Pediatrics, 21,* 48–51.

Smith, M. S., Mitchell, J., McCauley, E. A., & Calderon, R. (1990). Screening for anxiety and depression in an adolescent clinic. *Pediatrics, 85,* 262–266.

Society for Behavioral Pediatrics (SBP) Committee on Reimbursement. (1992). The breadth of developmental and behavioral services. *Journal of Developmental and Behavioral Pediatrics, 13,* 7–10.

Spinetta, J. J., & Maloney, L. J., (1978). The child with cancer: Patterns of communication and denial. *Journal of Consulting and Clinical Psychology, 46,* 1540–1541.

Stabler, B. (1979). Emerging models of psychologist–pediatrician liaison. *Journal of Pediatric Psychology, 4,* 307–313.

Stabler, B. (1988). Pediatric consultation-liaison. In D. K. Routh (Ed.), *Handbook of Pediatric Psychology* (pp. 538–566). New York: Guilford Press.

Stabler, B., & Mesibov, G. (1984). Role functions of pediatric and health psychologists in health care settings. *Professional Psychology, 15,* 142–151.

Stabler, B., & Murray, J. P. (1973). Pediatricians' perceptions of pediatric psychology. *Clinical Psychologist, 27,* 12–15.

Stabler, B., & Whitt, J. K. (1980). Pediatric psychology: Perspectives and training implications. *Journal of Pediatric Psychology, 5,* 245–251.

Stabler, B., Whitt, K., & Drotar, D. (1979, March). *Psychological consultation with physicians.* Workshop presented at annual meeting of the Southeastern Psychological Association. New Orleans, LA.

Stancin, T., Constantinou, G. M., & Walker, S. H. (1989). A regional consortium for behavioral pediatric education in residency programs. *Journal of Developmental and Behavioral Pediatrics, 10,* 147–150.

Stancin, T., Christopher, N., & Coury, D. (1990). Reported practices of pediatric residents in the management of attention deficit hyperactivity disorder. *American Journal of Diseases of Children, 144,* 1329–1333.

Starr, P. (1982). *Social Transformation of American Medicine.* New York: Basic Books.

Stein, R. E. K., & Jessop, D. J. (1991). Long-term mental health effects of a pediatric home care program. *Pediatrics, 88,* 490–496.

Stiffman, A. R., Earls, F., Robins, L., & Jung, G. (1988). Problems and help-seeking in high-risk adolescent patients of health clinics. *Journal of Adolescent Health Care, 9,* 305–309.

Strauss, M., Faberbaugh, S., Suczek, B., & Weiner, C. (1985). *Social Organization of Medical Work.* Chicago: University of Chicago Press.

Swedo, S. E., & Offer, D. (1991). The pediatrician's concept of the normal adolescent. *Journal of Adolescent Health, 12,* 6–12.

Takanishi, R. (1993). The opportunities of adolescence: Research, interventions, and policy. *American Psychologist, 48,* 85–87.

Tarnowski, K. J., (1991). Disadvantaged children and families in primary care settings: I. Broadening the scope of integrated mental health services. *Journal of Clinical Child Psychology, 20,* 351–359.

Tarnowski, K. J., Kelly, P. A., & Mendlowitz, D. K. (1987). Acceptability of behavioral pediatric interventions. *Journal of Consulting and Clinical Psychology, 55,* 435–436.

Task Force on Pediatric Education. (1978). *The Future of Pediatric Education.* Evanston, IL: American Academy of Pediatrics.

Tefft, B. M., & Simeonsson, R. J. (1979). Psychology and the creation of health care settings *Professional Psychology, 10,* 558–570.

Thompson, R. J., Jr. (1987). Psychologists in medical schools. Medical staff status and clinical privileges. *American Psychologist, 42,* 866–868.

Thompson, R. J., Jr. (1989). Child life programs in pediatric settings. *Infants and Young Children, 2,* 75–82.

Thompson, R. J., Jr. (1991). Psychology and the health care system. Characteristics and transactions. In J. J. Sweet, R. H. Rosensky, & S. M. Tovian (Eds.), *Handbook of Clinical Psychology in Medical Settings* (pp. 11–25). New York: Plenum Press.

Tomes, H. (1994, March). Health Security Act. Lacking in key areas. *APA Monitor, 25*(3), 40.

Tuma, J. M. (1982). *Handbook for the Practice of Pediatric Psychology.* New York: John Wiley & Sons.

Vane, J. R., & Demaria, T. (1988). The psychologist as general family practitioner. *Professional Psychology: Research & Practice, 19,* 118–120.

Varni, J. W., Katz, E. P., Colgrove, R., & Dolgin, M. (1992). The impact of social skills training on the adjustment of children with newly diagnosed cancer. *Journal of Pediatric Psychology, 18,* 751–767.

Walker, C. E. (1979). Behavioral intervention in a pediatric setting. In J. R. McNamara (Ed.), *Behavioral Approaches to Medicine: Application and Analysis* (pp. 227–266). New York: Plenum Press.

Walker, C. E., Milling, L. S., & Bonner, B. L. (1988). Incontinence disorders, enuresis, and encopresis. In D. K. Routh (Ed.), *Handbook of Pediatric Psychology* (pp. 363–399). New York: Plenum Press.

Wallander, J. L., Varni, J. W., Babani, C. B., & Wilcox, K. T. (1989). Disability parameters, chronic strains, and adaptation of physically handicapped children and their mothers. *Journal of Pediatric Psychology, 14,* 23–42.

Weithorn, L. A., & Campbell, S. B. (1982). The competency of children and adolescents to make informed treatment decisions. *Child Development, 33,* 1589–1598.

Weithorn, L. A., & McCabe, M. A. (1988). Emerging ethical and legal issues in pediatric psychology. In D. K. Routh (Ed.), *Handbook of Pediatric Psychology* (pp. 567–606). New York: Guilford Press.

Wender, E. H., & Friedman, S. B. (1985). Conference background and overview. *Journal of Developmental and Behavioral Pediatrics, 6,* 179.

Whitehead, W. E., & Schuster, M. M. (1985). *Gastrointestinal Disorders. Behavioral and Physiological Basis for Treatment.* New York: Academic Press.

Whitt, J. K., & Casey, P. H. (1982). The mother–infant relationship and infant development: The effect of pediatric intervention. *Child Development, 53,* 948–956.

Wilson, J. L. (1964). Growth and development of pediatrics. *Journal of Pediatrics, 65,* 984–991.

Wise, P. H., & Myers, A. (1988). Poverty and child health. *Pediatric Clinics of North America, 35,* 1169–1187.

Wright, L. (1967). The pediatric psychologist: A role model. *American Psychologist, 22,* 323–325.

Wright, L. (1985). Psychology and pediatrics: Prospects for cooperative efforts to promote child health—A discussion with Morris Green. *American Psychologist, 40,* 949–952.

Zaslow, M. J., & Takanishi, R. (1993). Priorities for research on adolescent development. *American Psychologist, 48,* 185–192.

Index

Access to care
  for economically disadvantaged children, 212
  in health care reform, 212
Administrative organization
  as obstacle to collaboration, 67
  as obstacle to pediatric psychology programs, 102–103
  in pediatric psychology programs, 106–114
  role of communication in, 106
Adolescent medicine
  Society of, 185
  training physicians in, 185–186, 188–192
  unique aspects of, 185–186
Adolescent medicine clinic
  clinical care in, 186–193
  collaboration in, 186–193
  consultation issues in, 186–193
  need for psychological services in, 185–186
  training physicians in, 185–186, 188–192
  training psychologists in, 189–190
Advocacy
  for children with chronic health conditions, 79, 84
  for sexually abused children, 46
  role of AAP in, 217–219
  role of APA in, 217–219
Alfred I. DuPont Institute Children's Hospital
  pediatric psychology at, 112–113
Ambulatory care: *see* Primary care
American Academy of Pediatrics (AAP)
  collaboration with APA, 20, 216–219
  current initiatives, 8
American Academy of Pediatrics (AAP) (*cont.*)
  formation of, 8
  liaison with Section on Clinical Child Psychology, 217
  liaison with Society of Pediatric Psychology, 217
  practice patterns of, 209–210
  report of Committee on Psychosocial Aspects of Child and Family Health (1993), 35
  role in legislation, 216–219
  Task Force on Coding for Mental Health in Children, 216–217
  Task Force on Pediatric Education (1978), 12
  workforce trends, 209–210
American Medical Association, 8, 210
American Pediatric Society, 8, 10
American Psychological Association (APA)
  collaboration with AAP, 20, 216–219
  efforts in medical education, 13
Anticipatory guidance, 43, 46–48
Archives of Pediatrics, 8
Arkansas Children's Hospital
  pediatric psychology at, 109–110
Attention-deficit disorder (ADD), 132
Attention-deficit hyperactivity disorder (ADHD), 36, 38, 45, 132–133, 188
  pediatric management of, 132–133

Behavioral methods
  evaluation of, 46–48, 138–141
  research on, 46–48, 138–141

Behavioral pediatrics
  Consortium of Northeastern Ohio, 153–154
  emergence of, 11–12
  First National Conference On, 12
  future trends, 210–212
  relationship to pediatric psychology, 211–212
  Society for, 12
  training in, 211
Behavioral problems
  pediatric identification of, 131–132
  pediatric management of, 132–134
  pediatric screening of, 131–132
  psychological intervention for, 138–141
Boston Children's Hospital, 90
Brief therapy
  in primary care settings, 43, 138–141

Cancer
  clinical services for, 77–78, 82–86
  comprehensive care for, 77–78, 82–86
  consultation in, 77–78, 82–86
  educational liaison in, 84–85
  family support in, 83–85
  parent support in, 83–85
  psychological evaluation in, 85
  research in, 85–87
  school consultation in, 85–86
Case conferences
  role in collaboration, 25, 58–63
Case review: *see* Collaborative case review
Case supervision
  in adolescent medicine, 188–189, 190–191
  in family medicine, 196
  of pediatricians, 39–40
Case Western Reserve University
  pediatric psychology training program, 147–148, 150–152
  training in collaborative research, 150–152
Child Abuse Prevention and Treatment Act, 219
Child life, 65
  collaboration with, 65
  role in program for childhood cancer, 84
  role in collaborative case review, 61
Child psychiatry
  collaboration with, 129
  pediatricians' perceptions of services, 130, 134–135
Children's Bureau, 8
Children's Hospital of Columbus
  pediatric psychology at, 111–112
Children's Hospital of Philadelphia
  Division of Oncology, 82–86
  psychosocial services at, 82–86
Children's Television Act of 1990, 218–219
Chronic health conditions in children
  barriers to services for, 75–77, 81–82
  collaborative management of, 75–87
  comprehensive care of, 77–87
  consultation for, 57–58, 77–79, 175–181
  ethical issues in care of, 79–80
  future needs of, 86–87
  interdisciplinary care of, 75–87
  intervention for, 77–78, 80–87
  parent education and support programs for, 84
  program development for, 82–87
  psychological services for, 77–78, 80–87, 175–181
  research concerning, 85–87
  school consultation for, 84–85
Chronic illness: *see* Chronic health conditions in children
Clarifying referral requests in primary care settings, 40
Clinical privileges
  for psychologists in hospitals, 126–127
Colitis
  psychological consultation for, 177, 181
Collaboration among psychologists and pediatricians, 1–4
  early developments in, 8–11, 13–16
  empirical studies of, 129–142
  ethical issues in, 117–127
  future of, 209–220
  history of pediatric inpatient settings, 49–64
  in pediatric psychology programs, 101–111
  in primary care settings, 35–38, 159–194
  in programs for children with chronic health conditions, 75–87
  in program development, 2, 106–111
  in research, 46–48
  in teaching, 38–40
  models of, 23–27, 38–40
  modern growth of, 16
  new opportunities for, 157–203

Collaboration among psychologists and pediatricians (*cont.*)
psychologists' views of, 15
professional issues in, 117–127
relationships in, viii, 22
research concerning, 127–142
role of communication in, 42–43, 55–56, 59–63, 101–102
training psychologists for, 143–155
See also Consultation, Interdisciplinary collaboration, Psychological consultation
Collaborative case reviews, 58–63
development of, 58
group problem solving in, 58–59
follow-up of, 59
implementation of, 58–61
liaison in, 61
promoting policy by, 61–62
role of other professions in, 59–62
teaching in, 62–63
Collaborative comprehensive care, 75–87
advocacy in, 79, 84
barriers to, 75–77, 79–80
clinical services in, 77–78, 80–82, 83–86
development of, 78–79
for children with chronic health conditions, 75–87
future needs for, 86–87
stresses of, 79–80
team functioning in, 78–79
See also Chronic health conditions in children
Collaborative practice of pediatric psychology, 44–46, 159–171
benefits of, 181–182
challenges of, 169–171
clinic location and structure, 160–161
clinical services in, 44–46, 164, 179–181
developing a, 159–171
developing referrals for, 165–167
early example of, 13
in community pediatric settings, 44–46, 159–171
in pediatric gastroenterology, 173–184
in primary care settings, 44–46, 159–171
legal and accounting issues in, 162–164, 184
marketing of, 165–166
models of, 77–82
Collaborative practice of pediatric psychology (*cont.*)
mutual learning in, 181–182
negotiation in, 160–161
of pediatric psychology, 44–46, 159–171
parents' perceptions of, 167–168
reimbursement and expenses in primary care settings, 85–48
research in, 46–48, 166
services in, 44–46, 164
setting up a, 160–164
Collaborative relationships
characteristics of, 22
development of, 205–206
stages of, 22
tensions in, 207–208
See also Collaboration, Interdisciplinary collaboration
Collaborative research, 89–100
advantages of, 89–93
future directions in, 98–100
future opportunities, 215–216
in primary care settings, 96–118
models of, 91–93
problems in, 96–98
role in program development, 99–100
securing resources and support for, 93–95
training in, 98–99
See also Research
Collaborative teaching
at a regional level, 153–155
development of, 12–15
early examples of, 12–15
future opportunities for, 215
support for, 153–155
See also Training
Communicating with hospital staff, 70–72
in inpatient settings, 53, 55–56
Communicating with physicians
in collaborative case reviews, 59–63
in developing pediatric psychology programs, 101–102
in inpatient settings, 55–56
in primary care, 42–43
See also Collaboration, Consultation, Psychological consultation
Compliance
enhancement of, 48
research concerning, 48

Compliance (*cont.*)
with consultation, 41
with medical care, 200
with psychological follow-up, 38
Conflicts
among psychologists, 104
among professionals, 67–70
in clinical management, 119–124
in collaboration, 67–70, 96–98
in patient care, 119–124
in professional boundaries, 67–70
in professional roles, 67–70
in research collaboration, 96–98
prevention of, 70–77
Confidentiality, 117–119
Consultation
client-centered, 23
collaborative team model, 26
consultee-centered, 23
independent functions model of, 23–24
indirect model of, 23–25
issues in adolescent medicine, 192–193
models of, 23–25
new opportunities for, 157–203
process-educative model of, 211–225
systems approach, 26–28, 57–58
training psychologists for, 143–155
with physicians other than pediatricians, 3
See also Collaboration, Interdisciplinary collaboration, Psychological consultation
Continuing education, 124
Fort Worth Children's Medical Center, 160
Crisis Intervention
in pediatric inpatient settings, 49
in primary care settings, 143
Crohn's disease, 173
Cystic fibrosis
consultation concerning, 61–62
psychological research in, 91, 95–96

Developmental pediatrics
emergence of, 11–13
Society for, 12
Developmental problems
pediatric identification of, 131–132
pediatric management of, 131–132
pediatric screening of, 131–132
Diabetes: *see* Insulin-dependent diabetes mellitus
Diagnostic and Statistical Manual of Mental Disorders (DSM), 131, 216–217
relation to Task Force on Coding for Mental Health in Children, 216–217

Empirical studies of consultation and collaboration, 129–142
Encopresis
psychological consultation for, 37, 173, 177
psychoeducational services for, 183–184
End-stage renal failure
collaboration in programs for, 78–80
consultation in programs for, 78–80
ethical issues in, 80
interdisciplinary collaboration in, 78–80
program development for, 78–80
Ethical issues
in care of children with chronic health conditions, 79
in collaboration, 112–127
in collaborative research, 89
in comprehensive care programs, 80
in consultation, 117–127
Evaluation
of brief targeted therapy, 138–140
of collaboration, 129–141
of consultation, 129,141
of psychological services in primary care, 46–48, 138–141

Failure to thrive (FTT)
clinical management of, 80–82, 99–100, 122, 178
collaborative management of, 80–82
consultation concerning, 54
research in, 72, 99–100
teaching about, 39, 62
Family medicine
activities of psychologists in, 195–203
biopsychosocial model in, 195
clinical services in, 197–202
collaboration in, 195–203
psychological consultation in, 195–203
role of behavioral science in, 195, 198–200
teaching physicians in, 197–203
training physicians in, 197–203
obstacles to collaboration in, 202–203
Family practice: *see* Family medicine

Feeding problems
psychological consultation for, 178
Fels Research Institute, 10
Fort Worth Pediatric Clinic
pediatric psychology services at, 160–164, 167
Future challenges: *see* Future directions of
Future directions of
collaboration with pediatricians, 209–221
collaborative practice, 171
consultation in adolescent medicine, 193–194
interdisciplinary collaboration, 72–73
pediatric practice, 209–214
pediatric psychology, 214–216
pediatric psychology programs in academic medical settings, 114–115
programs for children with chronic health conditions, 86–87
research on consultation, 141
research-related collaboration, 92–99
training in collaboration, 155
Future needs: *see* Future directions of

Guidelines
for clinical consultation in primary care, 40
for clarifying referral requests, 40, 51–52
for clinical consultation in inpatient settings, 51–54
for communicating with multiple staff, 53
for communicating with pediatricians, 40, 51–54
for discussing referrals with family members, 41, 53–54
for report writing, 42–43, 55–56
for structuring referral procedures, 40–41

Hassler Center for Family Medicine, 196
Health care reform, 212–214
impact on collaboration, 213–214
impact on psychological services, 213–214
impact on pediatric practice, 212
implications of, 212–214
role of collaborative practice in, 213–214
role of evaluation in, 213–214
role of managed care in, 213–214
Health maintenance organization
in collaborative practice, 164–170
Health Security Act of 1993: *see* Health Care Reform
HIV infection
psychological research in, 92–93, 152–153
Hospitalized children
guidelines for clinical consultation for, 51–54
identification of behavioral and developmental problems by pediatricians, 131–132

Independent functions model, 23–24
Indirect consultation model, 23–25
Inflammatory bowel disease, 173, 176–177
psychological consultation for, 176–177
Inpatient consultation
psychoeducational services for, 176–177
See also Collaboration, Consultation, Psychological Consultation, Inpatient Settings
Inpatient settings
collaboration in, 49–63
consultation in, 49–63
guidelines for consultation, 51–54
interdisciplinary communication in, 53, 55–62
referral problems in, 49–50
psychological services in, 49–50
teaching in, 62–63
Insulin-dependent diabetes mellitus (IDDM)
example of consultation in, 55–56
research in, 91, 96
Interdisciplinary collaboration
barriers to, 29, 67–70
beliefs and expectations concerning, 28–30
collaborative case reviews in, 58–61
commitment to, 70
definition, 19
dimensions of, 19–20
efficacy of, 29, 32–34
ethical issues in, 79, 117–127
future needs in, 32–33, 72–73
goals of, 19–20
implementation of, 70–72
incentives for, 29
influences on, 28–30
in adolescent medicine clinic, 187–188
in comprehensive care programs, 75–87

Interdisciplinary collaboration (*cont.*)
in managing chronic health conditions, 75–87
managing problems in, 72
need for, 1–3, 28, 65–67
obstacles to, 29, 67–70
outcomes of, 19–20, 22, 28–30
participants in, 19–21
in primary care settings, 35–48
problems in, 72
professional boundaries in, 69–70
professional cultures in, 67–70
professional issues in, 67–70
professional roles in, 28–30, 32
program development in, 71
quality of, 29, 33
research in, 33
role of work demands in, 21
settings in, 19–21
situational constraints in, 30–32
situational incentives in, 30–32
skills in, 28–29, 31
success in, 32–33
support for, 71–72

Jefferson Medical College, 112
Joint Commission on Accreditation of Health Care Organizations (JCAHO), 126
Journal of Developmental and Behavioral Pediatrics, 12

Laura Spellman Rockefeller Memorial Fund, 10
Leukemia
case review of, 60–61

Managed care
role in health care reform, 213–214
Maryland Department of Health and Mental Hygiene, 99
Massachusetts General Hospital, 15
Maternal & Child Health, Research Branch, Bureau of Health Care Delivery and Assistance
funding in behavioral pediatrics training, 211
funding in adolescent medicine, 186
research conference in behavioral pediatrics, 17

Medical schools
pediatric psychology in, 101–115
program development in, 101–115
psychologists on faculty in, 13–15
Medical settings
administrative issues in, 106–113
integrating psychology in, 200–207
program development in, 101–115
MetroHealth Medical Center
training pediatricians in, 39–40
training psychologists in, 147–148
Minneapolis Children's Medical Center, 27

National Child Abuse Coalition, 219
National Consortium for Child and Adolescent Mental Health Services, 219
National Institute of Child Health and Human Development, 17, 219
National Institutes of Health
sponsored research, 92
Nemours Foundation, 112
See also Alfred I. Dupont Institute
New York Hospital–Cornell Medical Center, 10
Noncompliance: *see* Compliance
Nursing
collaboration with, 57–62, 65
consultation with, 57–62, 65
satisfaction with psychological consultation, 136–137
"New morbidity," 12

Oncology
collaboration in, 77–78, 82–86
comprehensive care in, 77–78, 82–86
consultation in, 77–78, 82–86
program development in, 82–86
psychological services in, 77–78, 82–86
See also Cancer
Outcomes
definition of, 22
of collaboration, 19–20, 184
of psychological consultation, 19–20, 129–142, 184
Ohio State University
department of pediatrics in, 111–112
pediatric psychology at, 111–112
Oklahoma Health Sciences Center, 50

Parents' perceptions of pediatric psychology services, 138–141, 167–168
Pediatric gastroenterology
clinical services in, 173–184
collaborative psychological practice in, 173–184
psychological consultation in, 175–181
referral problems in, 173–181
Pediatric psychology
development of, 13–16
history of, 13–16
future challenges in, 209–220
programs, 101–111
research training in, 150–153
training in, 143–155
See also Consultation, Collaboration, Psychological consultation, Society of Pediatric Psychology
Pediatric rehabilitation hospital
consultation in, 50
Physicians' expectations
of collaboration, 28–33
of consultation, 28–33
of psychologists, 28–33
Physician satisfaction
with consultation, 135–138
with psychological consultation, 135–138
with psychological services, 135–138
Prevention
in pediatric care, 131–132
in primary care settings, 46–48, 138–141
of sexual abuse in primary care, 46
Primary care settings
behavioral interventions in, 46–48, 138–141
clarifying referral requests in, 40
collaborative practice in, 44–46, 159–184
communicating with pediatricians in, 43–44
consultation methods in, 40–44
discussing referrals with families in, 41–42
evaluation of psychological services in, 138–141
giving feedback to pediatricians in, 42–43
guidelines for consultation in, 40–44
in academic medical settings, 37–44
prevention in, 46–48, 138–141
referral problems in, 36–37
Primary care settings (*cont.*)
research in, 46–48, 138–141
service delivery in, 36–37
structuring referral procedures in, 40–41
teaching pediatricians in, 38–40
Process educative consultation model, 24–25
Professional autonomy
development in medical settings, 126–127
role of clinical privileges in, 126–127
Professional competence
enhancement of, 125–126
limits of, 124–125
role of clinical privileges in, 126–127
practicing within boundaries of, 125–126
professional culture as obstacle to collaboration, 67–68
strategies to enhance, 125–126
Professional development of psychologists in medical settings, 124-127
Professional issues
in collaboration, 67–70, 117–127
in consultation, 117–127
See also Ethical issues
Professional role
boundaries in patient care, 119–124
conflicts in, 69–70, 119–124
in comprehensive care programs, 78–79
in collaboration, 40–44, 54–58, 67–71, 78–79
in consultation, 40–44, 54–58
See also Professional competence
Program development
for children with chronic health conditions, 71, 77, 81–86
See also Programmatic collaboration
Programmatic collaboration, 101–111
administrative communication in, 106
administrative identity in, 114
administrative organization in, 102–103, 107–113
common themes in, 113–114
decision making in, 101–106
definition of, 101
development of resources for, 107
diversity of activities in, 107–113
diversity of funding sources in, 113–114
enhancing success in, 104–107
examples of, 107–113

Programmatic collaboration (*cont.*)
funding in, 103–104
future directions in, 114–115
group support in, 107
ingredients of successful, 104–107
leadership in, 106, 114
obstacles to, 101–104
problematic communication in, 101–102
resources for, 103–104
support for, 100–104
teamwork in, 107
Psychiatry
administration of pediatric psychology in departments of, 103–104
Psychological consultation
actions in, 54–57
activities in, 19–20
description of, 19–34, 129–130
effectiveness in, 222–224
empirical studies of, 127–142
ethical issues in, 117–120
evaluation of, 127–142
guidelines for, 40–44, 51–56
in adolescent medicine clinic, 185–194
in collaborative practice, 44–46, 160–172
in community pediatric practice, 44–46, 160–172
in family medicine, 195–203
in pediatric gastroenterology, 178–184
in pediatric inpatient settings, 49–64
in primary care settings, 35–48, 40–46, 138–141
in programs for children with chronic health conditions, 75–88
obstacles to, 28–34
personal attributes in, 223–225
physicians' satisfaction with, 135–138
referral for, 36–37, 40, 49–54, 175–181
training psychologists for, 143–155, 223
See also Collaboration, Consultation, Interdisciplinary Collaboration
Psychological evaluation/assessment
in primary care settings, 40–43
in inpatient consultation, 54–55
in oncology programs, 85
in pediatric gastroenterology, 175–181
Psychological services
acceptability of, 137–138
in inpatient settings, 49–64
in pediatric gastroenterology, 175–181
Psychological services (*cont.*)
in primary care settings, 36–38, 40–46, 138–141, 159–208
for children with chronic health conditions, 77–87
for children with chronic psychophysiologic problems, 80–82
physicians' satisfaction with, 135–138
utilization by physicians, 130–131
See also Psychological consultation
Psychophysiologic problems
collaboration in management of, 80–82
consultation in, 80–82
obstacles in management of, 80–82
Public policy
collaboration concerning, 217–219
role of AAP in, 217–219
role of APA in, 217–219

Rainbow Babies & Children's Hospital, 49, 95
research collaboration in, 95–96
Recurrent abdominal pain (RAP)
clinical management of, 133–134
psychological consultation for, 177, 179–180
Referral problems and services
in pediatric gastroenterology, 175–181
in pediatric inpatient settings, 49–51
in primary care settings, 36–37
Referral requests
clarifying with families, 41, 53–54
clarifying with staff, 40, 51–54
communicating with physicians about, 40, 51–54, 179
communicating with multiple staff about, 53
Renal disease: *see* End-stage renal failure
Report writing
example in primary care consultation, 42–43
example in inpatient consultation, 55–56
Research
in adolescent medicine clinic, 192
in childhood cancer, 85–87
in pediatric psychology programs, 107–113
in primary care settings, 46–48, 166, 182
in program development, 98–99
training pediatricians, 89–100, 150–153
See also Collaborative research, Research-related collaboration

Research-related collaboration
advantages of, 89–91, 96
developing programs of, 91–93
developing support for, 94–95
future directions in, 98–100
models of, 91–93
problems in, 96–98
role in program development, 99–100
securing resources for, 93–94
strategies of, 94–95
training in, 98–99, 150–153
Research training
for collaborative research, 150–153, 190
methods of, 150–153, 190
See also Research, Research-related collaboration

Screening
of behavioral problems by pediatricians, 131–132
of developmental problems by pediatricians, 131–132
Service delivery
in primary care academic medical settings, 37–38
Sexual abuse
services in primary care, 46
Sheppard-Towner Act, 8
Sidney Farber Cancer Institute, 77
Social work
collaboration with, 65–67, 70–72, 77–80
consultation with, 65–67, 70–72, 77–80
role in collaborative case review, 59–62
role in family medicine, 195
satisfaction with psychological consultation, 136–137
Society for Behavioral Pediatrics
committee on reimbursement, 210–211
committee on social concerns in, 222
formation of, 12
liaison with SPP, 12
National Conference on, 12
Society for Developmental Pediatrics
formation of, 12
Society for Research in Child Development
funding of, 10
Society of Adolescent Medicine, 185
Society of Pediatric Psychology (SPP)
founding of, 16
liaison with AAP, 217
Society of Pediatric Psychology (SPP) (*cont.*)
liaison with SBP, 22
research contribution awardees, 216
Stresses
in collaborative care of children with chronic health conditions, 79–80
Supervision
of adolescent medicine physicians, 188–189, 193–194
of pediatricians, 39–40
of psychologists, 145–148, 150–152
of training in consultation, 145–148
See also Training, Training pediatricians, Training psychologists in consultation and collaboration
Systems approach to consultation, 26–28, 57–58

Task Force on Coding for Mental Health in Children, 216–217
Task Force on Pediatric Education, 12
Teaching: *see* Supervision, Teaching pediatricians, Training, Training pediatricians,
Training psychologists
Teaching conferences
in consultation, 20, 24–25
in primary care, 41
Teaching pediatricians
in pediatric inpatient settings, 62–63
in primary care settings, 38–40
through case review, 62–63
See also Supervision, Training pediatricians, Training psychologists in consultation and collaboration
Training
in adolescent medicine, 185–186, 188–192
in family medicine, 197–203
in psychological consultation, 143–155
in pediatric psychology, 143,155
for collaboration, 143–155
for collaborative research, 14, 150–153, 190
See also Supervision, Training, Training pediatricians,
Training psychologists in consultation and collaboration
Training pediatricians
to identify behavioral problems, 38–40
to identify developmental problems, 38–40

Training pediatricians (*cont.*)
in collaboration, 31–33
in collaborative management, 31–33, 38–40
in primary care settings, 38–40
role of precepting in, 39–40
Training psychologists in consultation and collaboration, 143–155
common dilemmas for students, 148–150
in adolescent medicine clinic, 189–190
in administration, 115
in collaborative practice, 170–171
in inpatient settings, 145–146
in medical schools, 14–15
in primary care settings, 146–148
methods of, 143–155
role of collaborative mentorship in, 151, 152
role of faculty research, 151–152
role of observation in, 145–146, 150
role of clinical supervision in, 146
role of modeling in, 145–146, 150
role of training and support for faculty in, 144–145, 153–155
structures for, 144–145
Training psychologists in collaborative research, 150–153, 190
See also Research-related collaboration, Research training
Transplantation: *see* End stage renal failure

Ulcer disease
psychological consultation for, 177
Ulcerative Colitis, 173, 176
psychological consultation for, 180–181
University of Arkansas for Medical Sciences
department of pediatrics at, 109–110
pediatric psychology at, 109–116
University of Iowa
hospital school, 14
pediatric psychology training at, viii, 14
University of Iowa College of Medicine
department of pediatrics at, 108
pediatric psychology at, 108–109
University of Kansas, 47
University of Maryland Department of Pediatrics, Growth and Nutrition Clinic, 99
University of North Carolina School of Medicine, 45–46

William T. Grant Foundation, 11–12

Yale Child Study Center, 10
Yale Clinic for Child Development, 10

9 780306 484407